Green

MORNINGS OF JOY

Mornings of Joy

Pennie Kidd

KINGSWAY PUBLICATIONS
EASTBOURNE

First published 1987

ISBN 0 86065 417 6

Front cover photo: The Image Bank

Text illustrations by John Dillow

Printed in Great Britain for
KINGSWAY PUBLICATIONS LTD
Lottbridge Drove, Eastbourne, E. Sussex BN23 6NT by
Richard Clay Ltd, Bungay, Suffolk.
Typeset by CST, Eastbourne, E. Sussex.

This book is dedicated to
Maurice,
who knows, understands and loves.

AUTHOR'S NOTE:

To avoid the awkwardness of constantly repeating the phrase 'he or she' when referring to the baby, I have opted for 'he' in all cases. This is purely for reasons of simplicity. I have concentrated on a mother's first delivery, experienced in hospital, and have assumed the father would be present—realizing this may not always be possible or desired, and that some mothers choose a home confinement.

BY THE SAME AUTHOR:

I'm Smiling as Hard as I Can (Mowbray, 1981)
Learning about Christian Childbirth (booklet) (Mowbray, 1984)

Contents

Acknowledgements

I would like to thank Maurice, my husband, for his encouragement and his belief in this book. My boys Christopher, Tim and Jonathan for their patience and affection. My thanks also to Jane Watts for typing the script so willingly, to Sheila Roberts (tutor for the NCT) for checking the technical and medical details, and to Carole Derham (breastfeeding counsellor for the NCT) for help with the feeding chapter. Finally I wish to acknowledge Sheila Kitzinger, childbirth educator, and Harry Williams, theologian, who have been a constant inspiration to me through their written word.

Introduction

So much excellent material has been written on the subject of childbirth that it is with some trepidation I put pen to paper. Having a baby today is perhaps easier than it has ever been. Modern technology has made birth safer and now with the realization that technology should not take over the birth experience, but rather stay alongside in case of need, the young couple has a new freedom to relish the whole birth experience as naturally and as joyfully as possible.

I hope this book will not only inform couples about pregnancy and birth, but will add a further dimension. I believe that when two loves fuse together to begin a new life, there is the greatest miracle of all: the bonding of two persons which ultimately leads to the creation of a new individual made in the image of God. Surely there can be no greater privilege and joy for a young Christian couple than knowing that their love is taken up into the divine purpose and that they are so much a part of God's love that, deep inside the mother's body, God's creation is at work. As parents we are not merely empty vessels in which this miracle is occurring, we are joint heirs in Christ entering fully into the responsibility of, and caring for, the new baby even before conception. We can prayerfully prepare for pregnancy, birth and parenthood by ensuring we are enveloped by God's love. Showing love for one another and for ourselves brings discovery of the Spirit of Christ deep within our souls. There is little more beautiful than a young couple in love with each other, in love with God and in love with life. Here is the right medium for the growth of a new baby where, right from the start of his creation, the baby is saturated with love and care and the gentle touch of God.

Breathe on me, Breath of God,
Fill me with life anew;
That I may love what thou dost love
And do what thou wouldst do.

Edwin Hatch

Pregnancy and giving birth can be a time of deep spiritual renewal, yet in some Christian homes literature about having babies has been banished to a high bookshelf! I believe it should be brought into the very centre of our Christian experience and family life.

My husband, Maurice, and I have been privileged to give birth to three sons. Our love for the boys and for each other is the deepest experience of loving, and of being loved, that we have in this life—as it is for most parents. Yet our earthly love is but a pale reflection of God's love for each one of us. If this is how we love, how much more our heavenly Father loves, knows, weeps and rejoices with us as we journey on through life. My prayer is that all who share the joy and suffering of human birth may come to a lasting knowledge of God's love, and of his 'how much moreness' for them and their precious baby.

Meditation

O worship the Lord in the beauty of holiness,
Bow down before him, his glory proclaim;
With gold of obedience, and incense of lowliness,
Kneel and adore him, the Lord is his name.

Low at his feet lay thy burden of carefulness;
High on his heart he will bear it for thee,
Comfort thy sorrows and answer thy prayerfulness,
Guiding thy steps as may best for thee be.

Fear not to enter his courts in the slenderness
Of the poor wealth thou wouldst reckon as thine;
Truth in its beauty, and love in its tenderness,
These are the offerings to lay on his shrine.

These, though we bring them in trembling and
  fearfulness,
He will accept for the name that is dear;
Mornings of joy give for evenings of tearfulness,
Trust for our trembling, and hope for our fear.

O worship the Lord in the beauty of holiness,
Bow down before him, his glory proclaim;
With gold of obedience, and incense of lowliness,
Kneel and adore him, the Lord is his name.

John Samuel Bewley Monsell

CHAPTER ONE

The Beauty of Holiness

Emotional wholeness
Physical wholeness
Spiritual wholeness
Wholeness shared
Prayer

IF HOLINESS IS 'wholeness' it is beautiful. Wholeness is something we need to look at before we think further about pregnancy and birth. If we can be emotionally, physically and spiritually whole, then we are a step nearer to holiness. The beauty of holiness is something you can take with you through this journey of pregnancy and birth.

Emotional wholeness

When you come home and your husband calls out, 'Who is it?' so often you can find yourself saying, 'It's only me.' *Only* me! No, it's *me*. It is me who is loved, valued and cherished by God and by my partner! We need to be confident in ourselves, confident that we feel good inside. So often we have been brought up to feel that confidence will lead to pride and all sorts of pitfalls! When we are pregnant we especially need a glowing confidence that we are beautifully feminine, working *with* our rounded softened bodies, not pulling against the changes that are going on each day. If we are emotionally whole, we will be mature enough to relate to our parents as friends, no longer over-dependent on Mother for advice and guidance. We are whole enough to love and be loved by our partners, to accept our coming role as parents to our child.

Pregnancy is a time when it is natural to feel emotionally sensitive. Laughter can quickly be followed by tears; anger melts into joy. This is the beauty of the natural vulnerability of pregnancy. When you can smile through tear-filled eyes at the one who loves you, and find each other in that magic moment of togetherness and mutuality—that is wholeness. You are grown up enough to be child-like together. When you can share the dark fears that pregnancy sometimes holds—that is wholeness. Most mothers and fathers fear for the baby: will he be normal? Will he be all right? A chance remark by a tired obstetrician or midwife can bring fears. 'The baby is a little one', meant reassuringly, can cause you to worry that the baby has not developed enough. Almost any remark can quickly upset you, but being able to share these worries openly together is so valuable.

Sometimes couples are very close, yet there's still something preventing wholeness. I call it 'teasing down'. It can become such a part of your relationship that it casts a real shadow between you. It happens when there are constant jokes or teasing about each other that actually rob you of confidence and a sense of wellbeing. 'Sally's so big and fat she waddles like a pregnant duck!' or, 'Bill will never make a good dad, he doesn't know one end of a baby from the other!' You know what I mean. There comes a time for this teasing to cease. Be real together. If you're angry with each other, say so. Be honest and open. Teasing is so often a hidden aggression. Don't be afraid to have a healthy row over something, it's hardly ever as bad as you think and soon you will be making up, another step deeper in love, and you feel good inside again.

This feeling inside is so important. When children have grown up without demonstrative love, affection and praise, they can feel an emptiness, or even a badness inside.

Then comes the question: 'Can anything so good as a perfect baby come out of me?' and thus follow all the fears about the baby and guilt about your fears and depression because of your guilt! We need to see ourselves as whole, confident in ourselves as secure people who love and are lovable. We need to feel the pleasure of our pregnancy for ourselves and for each other. You're not pregnant just to please Grandma, or to fulfil the expectations of friends, family or society. You're pregnant so that you can revel in the delights of being expectant parents together for yourselves and your baby, and the growing love that is between you and all that is so pleasing to God.

Physical wholeness

Being healthy is half the battle, so they say. Many mums experience radiant health while they are pregnant. Even if they've felt a bit under the weather in the first three months, the middle months can be especially good.

But why is it only half the battle? I believe that even if you are not particularly healthy physically, it is your attitude that is so vital. Pregnancy is a time when all sorts of people are interested in your body. This can feel like a real invasion of your privacy. The very fact of being pregnant is the outward sign that you have had sexual intercourse! Your body is no longer your own personal affair. Midwives will prod you, weigh you, listen to your baby's heartbeat. Doctors will examine you, take samples of blood and urine to test, and take sonic pictures (scans) of your baby. How do you feel about all this?

Again, you need to feel good physically. You need to make friends with your body and to accept its changes, its new beauty and its aches and pains! You need to know deep down inside that your body is perfectly designed to give birth. Your body is capable and you are confident. It will help you to accept your body if you understand all that is happening to you. This is one good reason to go to classes together to prepare for childbirth, and to read books on the subject. To understand is to eliminate so much fear of the unknown. Through pregnancy and birth you will need to learn to relax your body and to be in tune with your body. So often a 'tight' Christian upbringing, with all its sense of guilt over anything sexual, brings with it a tight or stiff upper lip attitude to pain, or pleasure, and with it a tight birth canal, tight breathing, tight muscles. 'Tense' is a better word, but 'tight' can reflect the moral and social tightness of our upbringing and culture. Somehow British girls feel they have neat little bodies and neat little vaginas, whereas the Mediterranean cultures are more effusive and may do better in childbirth because of it. 'Cleanliness is next to godliness' is another old favourite—and the thought of birth being a messy, earthy, natural affair can be alarming to our clean, disinfected selves. We need to relax, accept our bodies as good friends, and treat our bodies lovingly. When you are tired, rest. When you hurt, nurse yourself and your partner. There is a natural tenderness which comes with love and this tenderness reflects your emotional and physical wholeness. There need never be a taboo on tenderness, but rather a delight in its sensitivity and grace.

Spiritual wholeness

Spiritual wholeness begins when we can learn to accept our humanity. So often I feel people seek God 'out there', somewhere distant and high, as though he were hanging around the solar system! He is totally involved with our humanity. Our acceptance of our physical, emotional, earthy being, with all its wonder and complexities, is the beginning of self-awareness. Our acceptance of pregnancy with all of its physical and sexual aspects, and the acceptance of our more difficult or damaged relationships with those close to us, can be like a cross which leads us to a resurrection with Christ. We share 'the power of his resurrection, and the fellowship of his sufferings' (Philippians 3:10). Our burden is looking into the dark places, and the richness of joy is finding Christ there, already in us, waiting for us to realize it and acknowledge him. If we avoid facing our human lot, that bad feeling hidden away deep within ourselves, we resist our attempt at self-awareness, of Christ-awareness, which is the prerequisite of self-acceptance. Once we can look this dark part of us in the face, it loses its power over us, loses its hold, we discover a new freedom and wholeness as the darkness fades and the light and warmth of Christ gently unfolds within our being. Our personalities are made more wholesome, and we have taken another step towards a deeper relationship with God. Often we have been taught to deny ourselves, to cross ourselves out: like a cross is 'not I, but I crossed out'. I believe this self denial is a denial of Christ's gospel. We end up being proud of being nothing, proud of being empty, proud of being humble! Rather we should let God enhance our value, and we should renounce all that devalues us! We discover in the adventure of opening ourselves up to God that we find new life.

> Love is the consciousness of self survival in the act of self surrender.
>
> *Nettleship*

It is really an adventure with the love of God. With him we can accept our bodies, our animal selves, our sexual selves, our frightened selves. We rejoice in his unbelievable grace. Filled with his love we can feel confident, self-assured and ready to journey on through pregnancy, birth and on into life more abundant.

> Finally, brethren, whatsoever things are true, whatsoever things are honest, whatsoever things are just, whatsoever things are pure, whatsoever things are lovely, whatsoever things are of good report; if there be any virtue, and if there be any praise, think on these things (Philippians 4:8).

Wholeness shared

Growing in relationships is a happy/sad affair. There is the joy of new experience, but also the loss of past discoveries, of sureties and certainties. There is the anxiety and excitement of the future, the unknown, and the moving on from established patterns of life. You may not have been married for long before you both become pregnant. I say 'both', because it can be a totally shared experience of togetherness. Perhaps you still think back to your honeymoon when you could be carefree in your love, when bodies were slim and beautiful, where there was almost nothing between you in your love for one another. Now, perhaps before you've had time to explore your marriage further, and while you are still adjusting to one another as husband and wife, a child is expected and the changes involved for both of you can be challenging or even a little threatening.

It is just as well pregnancy takes nine long months, because although this can be physically tiring, it does allow time and space for both of you to be able to grow gradually into parenthood. Not only does the mother need to accept the changes that are occurring, but the new father needs to be, and feel, fully involved in the pregnancy. He may have almost no knowledge about childbirth, or maybe only a few odd notions gleaned through his boyhood. Ignorance inevitably leads to fear. Now is the time for you to commit yourselves to one another, to this pregnancy, to your new baby, and to commit the whole process to God. It would be wise to seek out help and to attend antenatal classes at your local hospital or clinic.

The National Childbirth Trust also run antenatal classes throughout the country. These classes consist of a small number of couples who not only learn in detail about the physical side of pregnancy and labour, but can also share their thoughts and feelings about the changes that are taking place, and about decisions that need to be made. The classes also give the opportunity to make real friends with other couples who live near you and much can be gained from these friendships.

One of the decisions of pregnancy is where to have your baby: at home or in hospital, and how long to stay in hospital if that is your choice. Nearly all mothers decide to have their babies in hospital where there is expert medical help at hand should they or their babies need it. Doctors these days are very reluctant to let a first-time mum have her baby at home, and if there is any type of medical problem you will need to be in hospital. It is possible, with the co-operation of your general practitioner and your local midwife, to arrange a 'domino' delivery. This means your midwife and your own doctor supervise your antenatal care. When labour starts, you usually go into hospital with your midwife. She delivers your baby in the hospital, but should you need extra help the hospital facilities are close by. When your baby is born, providing you are both fit and well, you will be allowed home after just a few hours of rest. Your midwife will then care for you at home. In many ways this is an ideal 'best of both worlds' situation. On the other hand you may especially want a home delivery. As this can be difficult to arrange, it may be helpful to contact the Society to Support Home Confinements, 17 Laburnham Avenue, Durham.

I have already mentioned how helpful it is to share your pregnancy, and this will mean both of you helping the other to accept and understand the physical, emotional and spiritual needs of one another. A new dad can feel almost cut off from his wife as she now seems to belong to the hospital, midwife or doctor. Strange words are written on cards about her and the baby, and this whole new antenatal world may suggest that men are not really welcome. Take my word for it, this is a time when Father is needed more than ever. His presence with his wife at antenatal clinics, when seeing a consultant or having a scan can be so reassuring. She may have lots of questions to ask the doctor or midwife, but seems to dry up or get it all wrong on the day of her appointment. If you are both there you can gently help one another to ask those questions. Should you not understand something that is said or written, you can ask immediately instead of coming home worried or upset. If you go to antenatal classes together you will be able to learn so much of interest, see films of birth, look around the labour ward, and you'll have so much to talk about when you get home.

As you both feel Baby kicking, you can wonder together about the future, share your excitement or your fears. You may have a name for the baby before he is born, perhaps it is a secret, intimate name you share together. You may find little things upset you, or you feel angry with each other. If you can cry and talk together you will grow through these difficult times, and learn from them.

There is nothing wrong with tears; it is not weak or silly to cry. You may cry at the very thought of your new baby, with the sheer wonder of it all, or cry from the frustrations of your limited ability to take part in the normal activities of life. You may worry for the baby, or get irritable with each other. All this is so normal in pregnancy. It is partly due to hormonal changes in the mother, but also a reaction in both of you to the great emotional upheavals, fears and excitements for the future. You can pray at these times. Perhaps you might like to put your hands over Baby, and come close, the three of you together, bringing yourselves into Christ's healing and comforting love for you all, then you can feel his blessing on you, and let go of all the tension, tiredness and tears. Just be you alongside him. There's no need to be formal over prayer. He is your friend. I like the prayers that begin, 'Hallo, Lord, it's me . . . .'

Dear Lord, we come to you
Full of wonder, full of praise.
Take our souls and bodies
That we may be taken up
In your love and made whole.
Bless us with your strength in our weakness,
And your love in our fear.
We come before you in warmth and
  tenderness
And pray for the blessing of a child.
May we become a family for you
Where love abounds in freedom and peace.
In the name of Jesus Christ our Lord.
Amen.

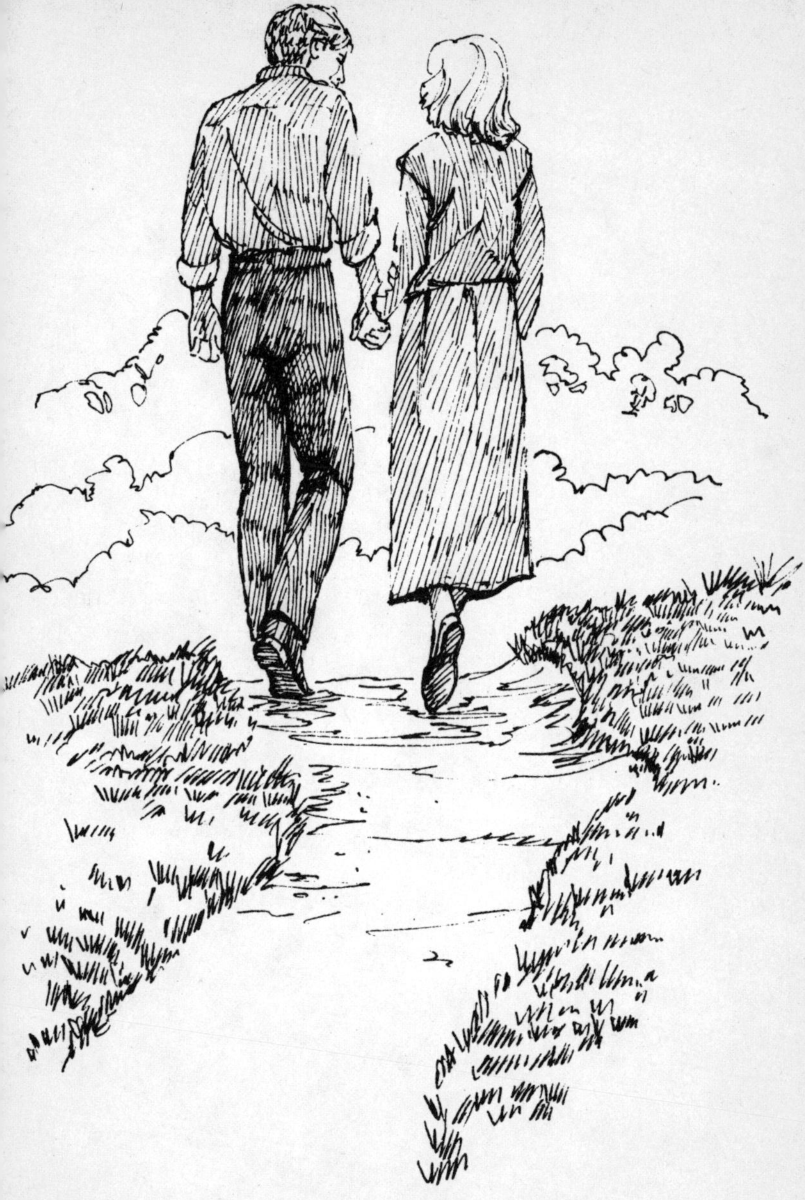

May we become a family for you.

CHAPTER TWO

His Glory Proclaim

Preparing yourselves
Pregnancy confirmed
The child within
Your baby's world
Prayer

Preparing yourselves

JESUS TELLS US to 'love your neighbour as yourself'. The first part of this command is often easier to obey than the second! So often Christians have sought to love their neighbours while actually denigrating themselves. We have already seen the importance of wholeness and I am utterly convinced that people who have had good, or at least 'good enough' mothering, develop into confident, lovable, loving mothers and fathers themselves. Girls and boys who know they are loved because they have seen, heard and felt their parents' love for them and for each other, over their entire lives, will discover a healthy love for their bodies and their innermost selves. When we love and respect ourselves, our minds and our bodies; when we acknowledge this love is from God and of God, then we are ready to become a vehicle for God's creation. We are ready to become parents to a new aspect of God, a new baby.

But what if you don't feel free to love yourself and your body? Well, let's start by looking at ourselves and our relationships. Have your parents openly praised you, shown you their non-possessive love and warmth? Now you can ask God to show you his love for you, maybe through your partner, or alone. Begin to think positively about yourself. You are loved. Lovable. Yes, you are treasured and cherished as yourself by our heavenly Father. Say it over to yourself several times, in prayer: 'I am loved and treasured and cherished.' As a young couple, preparing for your first child, say it to one another. You will find a new love deep down inside you and that love is a new experience of God. You will want to cry out your love for God. Share it together, let it flow through your lives and let it flow through you as your baby is conceived. How beautiful for your child to be conceived in pure godly love.

Don't put the sexual act to one side, as if a little embarrassed by it being 'not quite proper'! No, the union of two children of God is designed to be beautiful and pleasurable, both physically and spiritually. It binds us together within God's great love. From it is created God's greatest gift, God's expression of his love for us—a new baby, made in his own image. What a privilege. What a joy! What immense humility is felt as we try to grasp the reality of it all.

> Praise to the Holiest in the height,
> And in the depth be praise;
> In all his words most wonderful,
> Most sure in all his ways.
>
> *John Henry Newman*

Pregnancy confirmed

Perhaps you both long for a baby, or maybe you're not really sure. You may wonder whether you are expecting a baby or not. You may feel different as soon as you have conceived or it may be a surprise when you miss a period and you begin to think when your next period is due. If you miss a period and suspect that you are pregnant, it is a wise move to have the pregnancy confirmed. Not only will you have more peace of mind, but you will be able to start to care for yourself and your baby.

If you visit your family doctor two weeks or more after your last missed period, he will be able to test whether you are pregnant or not by sending off a sample of urine to a laboratory. Once you become pregnant there are hormonal changes which take place in your body and the urine test shows whether these hormones are there or not. A quicker result may be obtained by taking a sample of urine to a chemist that advertises pregnancy testing, or even by buying a pregnancy-testing kit. That way you can know the result within two hours. You may wish to test again a week later to be quite sure, followed by a visit to your doctor who will then check your general health and discuss the pregnancy with you, and give you an estimated date when your baby is due.

There are some very early signs of pregnancy which you may become aware of in your body. Your breasts may become fuller and a little tender. The dark area, called the areola, around your nipples may become darker, and the oil glands that keep the skin soft may stand out a little like goose pimples around the edge of the areola. You may feel tired and need to rest a lot. Your body is undergoing wonderful changes as it adapts to the new baby growing deep inside. It is not surprising that you need to rest a lot.

You may find that you feel slightly nauseated, or that you are sick at certain times of the day—often in the early morning. This is simply your body's reaction to the different hormones and you need not worry about it, unless of course it becomes severe, then you should see your doctor. Sometimes a piece of dry toast or a biscuit or two with a cup of tea, taken in bed before you get up, can be all that is needed to make you feel better.

Once you know you are expecting a baby you may be very excited, thrilled-to-bits, relieved or anxious. There may be a feeling of 'no turning back now' which can be a bit daunting! You have begun an exciting, tiring, wonderful and sometimes worrying journey. You may not feel ready to become parents, or you may rejoice that this privilege has come to you at this time. Either way I'm sure it is helpful to talk about these feelings together. Don't forget that Dad has lots of thoughts and feelings at this time too, and to talk things over together is good. You may want to keep it a secret between you for a while, a wonderful secret almost too precious to share, or you may want to tell the whole world that you are pregnant because you feel like the first people ever to be expecting a baby! I think that 'sharing' is a key word in pregnancy and childbirth. Now is the time to share your emotions, your thoughts and your bodies with each other as you get used to the idea, and indeed the reality, that your baby is growing deep in the mother's body. It is good for Mum to be aware of her new softness, roundness and tenderness as a woman, and for Dad to feel strong and supportive beside her. Both of you may have worries. Will you cope as parents? Will Baby be all right? Will you cope with the birth? All these thoughts are completely normal at this time. Share them together, and share them with God. Let him come into the joys and the worries, the laughter and the tears with you. You can trust him and lean on him, letting him hold you like a delicate bird's egg is held in the palm of the hand—not too firmly, not too softly, but gently cradling you so you never fall yet have the freedom to be yourselves.

The child within

By the time you know for certain that you are pregnant, your baby will have already undergone incredible development and growth. Once the tiny egg which has been released from the mother's ovary has been penetrated by a sperm, it starts to multiply. The cells divide into two, four, eight, sixteen, and so on, forming a little cluster of cells which journey down the fallopian tube and into the uterus. This journey takes as long as five to seven days. Once in the uterus, this cluster of cells, known as a blastocyst, fixes itself into the lining of the uterus which is rich in blood and nutriment. As the blastocyst nestles deep in the warm protective lining of the uterus, it is developing and organizing itself into different sets of cells which will form different structures.

So by the third week, and you may have just missed your period by now, there is the formation of a head, body and tail, all attached to a yolk sac. By the time you are six weeks' pregnant the blastocyst has become an embryo and, incredibly, it has a rudimentary working body with eyes, ears, brain and beating heart. It is now about the size of a peanut! Each day important developments take place. When you understand how quickly the embryo develops you will see how vital it is that you don't take any medicines or drugs unless prescribed by a doctor. Smoking, drinking and X-rays could retard the natural growth of the embryo at this stage.

By only eight weeks the embryo is formed and obviously human. The brain controls the functioning of the organs. Even the fingers and thumbs have fingerprints at this stage! Simple movements are made, although you will be quite unaware of them.

There is such a complicated development over these first eight weeks of life that it seems almost too incredible to be true. Yet it is all happening, the actual miracle of creation, God at work now, today, inside you! In a way, such a complicated and intricate piece of work is worrying and you can easily be anxious. It is a time to be sensible and caring towards yourself and to trust in the Lord and wait upon him. He will perform the great miracle and you need not be anxious. It can be a time of quiet prayer and meditation. A time to soak yourself in God's gentle warmth—like sunbathing on a beautiful summer's day. Bask in his light and love, and let it flow through you and your baby.

By twelve weeks the embryo is called a foetus. All the organs are complete—even if not yet very sophisticated. The baby can clench his fists, frown, even suck his thumb! He swallows the fluid he is floating in and passes it out through his bladder. At this stage, the all-important placenta begins to function and blood circulates between the baby and the placenta via the umbilical cord. It is in the placenta that nourishment and waste products, oxygen and carbon dioxide, are exchanged through a type of membrane.

At sixteen weeks you may begin to feel movements like butterflies low down in your abdomen, though it is quite normal to feel these early movements a little later. By twenty weeks the baby weighs about eight ounces and is about ten inches long. He is covered in a fine downy hair called lanugo. Hair grows on the head and eyebrows, and tiny fingernails develop. Soon the baby is covered in a greasy substance called vernix. This is a waterproof protection and some babies are born still streaked with vernix—it's a bit like the grease channel swimmers cover themselves with! At twenty-four weeks, although all limbs are the right proportion, there is very little fatty tissue.

Twenty-eight weeks marks a milestone in the pregnancy because it is at this time that the baby is 'legally viable'. There is a good chance of the baby surviving (with intensive medical and nursing care) if he is born at this time. Baby is active now, and you and Baby's brothers or sisters, if he is not the first baby, can enjoy seeing the movements on Mum's tummy as he wriggles around or kicks. It becomes a little easier to realize there really is a baby in there! From now on there is more growth, more fatty tissue is laid down and Baby looks more and more like the little bundle you will soon hold.

As Baby takes up more space in the ever-expanding muscular uterus, so his more vigorous kicking will feel much stronger, almost uncomfortable at times as he suddenly prods you hard under your ribs! To some mums it's all a little alarming, but it is also good and reassuring to know Baby is active and energetic. Once you come to thirty-six weeks, the baby may drop down a little in your abdomen. What is actually happening is that sometime between thirty-six and forty weeks the baby's head enters into the base of your pelvis ready to be born. The doctors and midwives will explain that the head is engaged. It gives you a little more space under your ribs, but the baby now presses more on your bladder so you will need to visit the toilet fairly frequently. Baby will now weigh something between five and eleven pounds and will be between eighteen and twenty-two inches long. He is beautifully developed, strong and ready for his birthday!

Your baby's world

We've looked at how your baby grows and develops while he is tucked up inside you, but what do we know of his experience deep in the womb? In China and Japan the baby is considered to be one year old when he is born because he has already had almost a year of life in the womb. Obviously not a great amount is known, but research has shown that the baby reacts to sound and light. The uterus is rather a noisy place! There is the constant whooshing sound of the mother's pulse with blood flowing along the arteries. Then there are rumbling sounds as air moves around the mother's intestines. Any external sounds, like music or voices, are muted against this constant pulse-beat. No wonder, when baby is born, he can be soothed by being held and rocked close to your heart where he will once again hear that reassuring heart-beat. If the baby in the uterus is disturbed by extra sound he will react with movement. He will also move in response to being touched through pressure on the abdominal wall. He may suck his thumb for comfort. Later in the baby's development, the eyes react to light. Light on the abdominal wall will cause a pink diffused light inside the uterus. Some studies have shown that if the mother is under severe emotional stress, then there is increased activity of the baby in the uterus and also after birth with more crying. All this means it's possible that Mother's anxiety is some-how transferred to Baby who also becomes more anxious. So your baby's world is one of being gently rocked as you walk around. It is rather noisy, with the constant but reassuring sound of your heartbeat, and it is warm, wet and slightly pink! Perhaps it's a little bit of heaven before he starts his journey through life!

I think it is delightful for Mum, Dad and Baby if they can get to know each other a little before birth. Get used to talking to your baby, 'hold' your baby and even sing to him. You'll soon learn what he enjoys! When you really relax and rest, you may find Baby starts a play time. The relaxation of the abdominal wall has given him a little more space to move around in, so he has a stretch. While you are busy walking or working, your movements are more likely to send him off to sleep.

You can wrap Baby in your love as you both feel him moving. It can be a wonderful time, full of secret delight. If you go to church and receive bread and wine at Holy Communion, remember you are taking Baby along with you. Offer yourselves and Baby into God's perfect peace and trust and, ever childlike, trust in him. He knows your innermost joys, your innermost fears, and he holds and supports you through this delicate sensitive time.

Throughout the pregnancy, starting with conception, you are in the privileged position of being able to pray for your unborn child. Couples may like to gently place their hands on the mother's abdomen and pray together. To surround your baby prayerfully in love can only bring good. You may give thanks that your baby is loved and has been given the gift of life. You may like to give thanks for your baby's growth and development, and as the weeks go by to pray for comfort and protection in the womb. Before the birth you can pray that birth will hold no fears for Baby, and that he will be able to accept the trauma of pressure and change, and that God's healing power will overcome any pain or shock that he may experience.

There is a blessedness of birth, and a blessedness of being. Surrounding your child with prayer will surely invite that blessedness which comes to us through him who experienced human birth in Bethlehem.

Lord, look with loving kindness
On this your child, as yet unborn.
May your creative love surround and
Protect this babe, held deep within,
That he or she may be filled with
Your heavenly blessing and grow in
Your fullness, to reflect your perfect image.
We thank you for this little one,
And pray that we may be worthy
Of that special privilege of care
As we journey through these coming
months.
We ask this in your name. Amen.

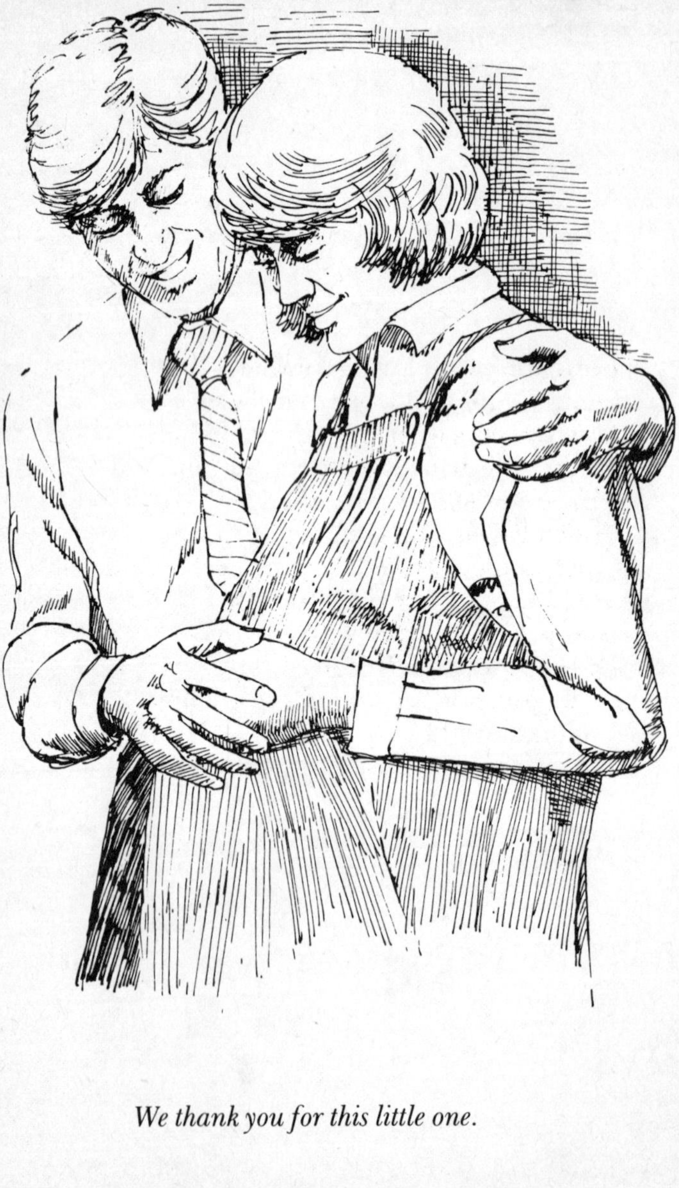

We thank you for this little one.

CHAPTER THREE

A Burden of Carefulness

WHAT A BEAUTIFUL way to describe your pregnancy: 'A burden of carefulness.' Yes, in so many ways it is a burden, a responsibility, as well as a privilege to care for yourselves and for your growing baby. Yet it is a burden God shares with you; it is a mutuality of carefulness.

> Come unto me, all ye that labour and are heavy laden, and I will give you rest. Take my yoke upon you, and learn of me; for I am meek and lowly in heart: and ye shall find rest unto your souls. For my yoke is easy, and my burden is light (Matthew 11:28-30).

Your body

If you understand how your body is made up and how it moves and works, you will learn how to care for it throughout pregnancy.

Think of the uterus, the bag your baby is tucked up in. It is strong and elastic, being made up of many layers of muscle. As the baby grows, so the uterus grows to accommodate the baby. At its base is the cervix, a firm neck with a canal running through the centre. This canal is blocked during the pregnancy with mucus, thus keeping the inside of the uterus quite safe. The cervix dips down into the top of your vagina. It feels like the tip of your nose, quite firm, until you are ready to give birth, when the cervix will become soft. The vagina is very stretchy—the soft, elastic, muscular walls form fan-like convolutions which will stretch out around your baby as it passes through at birth. Now this uterus, which becomes increasingly heavy needs to be held and supported by some firm bones. Your body has the perfect answer: a large bony cradle called your pelvis, or hips. The uterus is cradled deep in your pelvis, and as the baby grows so it expands and rises up out of the pelvis, but its weight is still held by these strong bones. Your pelvis is rather special as it not only holds the uterus but also supports your spine, and all the other abdominal organs. Just think of the weight put on your spine as the baby grows.

That brings me on to balance and how you walk and stand. Your spine and pelvis are quite able to cope with the extra weight, but you will strain your back if you are not well balanced. If you lean back to pull against the extra weight in front, or if you lean forwards over your bump, you will cause tension, strain and pain in your back. Try standing up, shoulders down and your tail tucked in. Think of something hanging just above you that you are trying to touch with your head. You will find your neck nicely stretching out, your chin tucked in, and your back straight. Practise this and feel like a model in a fashion show! You will also need to practise this balance after your baby is born when you push him around in a pram for a couple of years!

Now you may not realize that your pelvis is not only firm and strong, but it can rotate as well. Girls doing hoola-hoop movements, or belly dancing, are actually rotating the pelvis. It is very useful to practise rocking your pelvis in pregnancy. 'Pelvic rocking' as it is called keeps the ligaments around the bones supple, and if you do get any backache this will often ease it away. Try tucking your tail in, then out, and feel your pelvis rocking to and fro. Then try a round movement or a sideways swing. You can do this with your partner and enjoy it! This pelvic movement can be most helpful when you are in labour, but more of that later.

One more important aspect of your pelvis is the pelvic floor, or outlet, between your legs. This floor is actually made up of strong bands of muscle around your vagina and anus. Bands of muscle also run across and down. These muscles help to hold up the weight of the uterus and abdomen. When your baby passes out through the vagina, the muscles fan out and thin, and ease gently around your baby's head. If you are aware of these muscles and the way they can tighten up or relax, it will help you as you have your baby. Once Baby is born, these bands of muscle need to be toned up again to regain their full strength.

Try this pelvic floor exercise. Pretend your pelvic floor (also called perineum) is a lift in a shop! Pull the muscles up to the first floor, up again to the second floor, hold it a moment, then gently down to first floor, back to ground floor, then down to the basement (really relax) then always to finish back up to ground level again. Go on, no one will know you are doing your exercises. Do them at a bus stop, or each time you stop at traffic lights, or each time you wash up. It is a very important exercise and one you need to do several times a day for the rest of your life, so preventing prolapse problems when you are older. I tell my classes, it's no longer: 'Hallo, darling, have you had a nice day?' but: 'Hallo, darling, have you done your pelvic floor exercises?'!

Remember God has given you a wonderful body designed to carry a baby inside for nine months, and designed to open up and let the baby pass through into the world. But he needs your co-operation to keep your body fit and well. You need to play your part in your 'burden of carefulness', and you will discover that the 'burden' is a delight and a joy as you help one another through the coming months.

Caring for yourself

1. Diet

Isn't it strange how your body is your own until you are pregnant! Suddenly the lady next door, the family and even the greengrocer is telling you what to eat and how to look after yourself. One lady used to call across the road to me when I was very pregnant for the third time: 'Keep drinking the milk stout!'

However, diet *is* very important because your baby grows and develops on what you eat and drink. If you have steak and chips, your baby has steak and chips; if you starve, your baby starves. One phrase is useful to remember: 'More protein, less carbohydrates.'

You get more protein in lean meat, fish, beans, milk, cheese, butter and nuts. You need a generous helping of protein each day. 'High fibre' is all the rage these days, but it simply means bulk to help keep you healthy and active inside, and to prevent constipation. Bulk is obtained from cereals, wholemeal bread, fresh fruit and vegetables. You need at least one generous helping of these each day to add to your protein. If you eat the protein and fruit and vegetables you will also be getting the essential vitamins you and your baby need, and the extra calcium so necessary for the early development of strong, healthy teeth. Iron is another mineral essential for you both. It helps form the red blood cells which carry oxygen through your body. Iron is found in liver, egg yolk, dark vegetables (like spinach), nuts and raisins. Vitamin C helps the absorption of iron and is found in fresh vegetables and fruit, especially oranges.

Too many carbohydrates will cause you to put on extra unnecessary weight which if you're overweight to begin with may cause you problems in later pregnancy. Foods which contain lots of sugar should be avoided, like cakes, chocolate, puddings and sweets. As carbohydrates give you energy they are needed, but in moderation. A baked potato, wholemeal bread and cereals all contain carbohydrates which will provide the energy you need for yourself and your baby. If you understand calories, you only need an extra 200 calories per day. Your diet should be thought about carefully. You may be prescribed extra iron if your doctor feels you need more than you are getting through your diet.

2. Rest

To rest can be a lovely experience. Your body and your mind may become very tired. The early months especially seem to make huge demands on you, and towards the end of the pregnancy your body can become strained from the sheer weight you are carrying around. Telling you to sit down with your feet up, or to go to bed for an hour or so during the day is not enough unless you feel good about doing it. You may resent having to rest and rather angrily sit with your feet up, but this won't relieve the tension in your body and it won't be restful.

I like to link the word 'rest' with 'pray'. Not to work hard saying formal prayers, but just to rest in God's peace and grace, to feel totally supported by his arms, to smile and feel loved—as you love your baby. This is

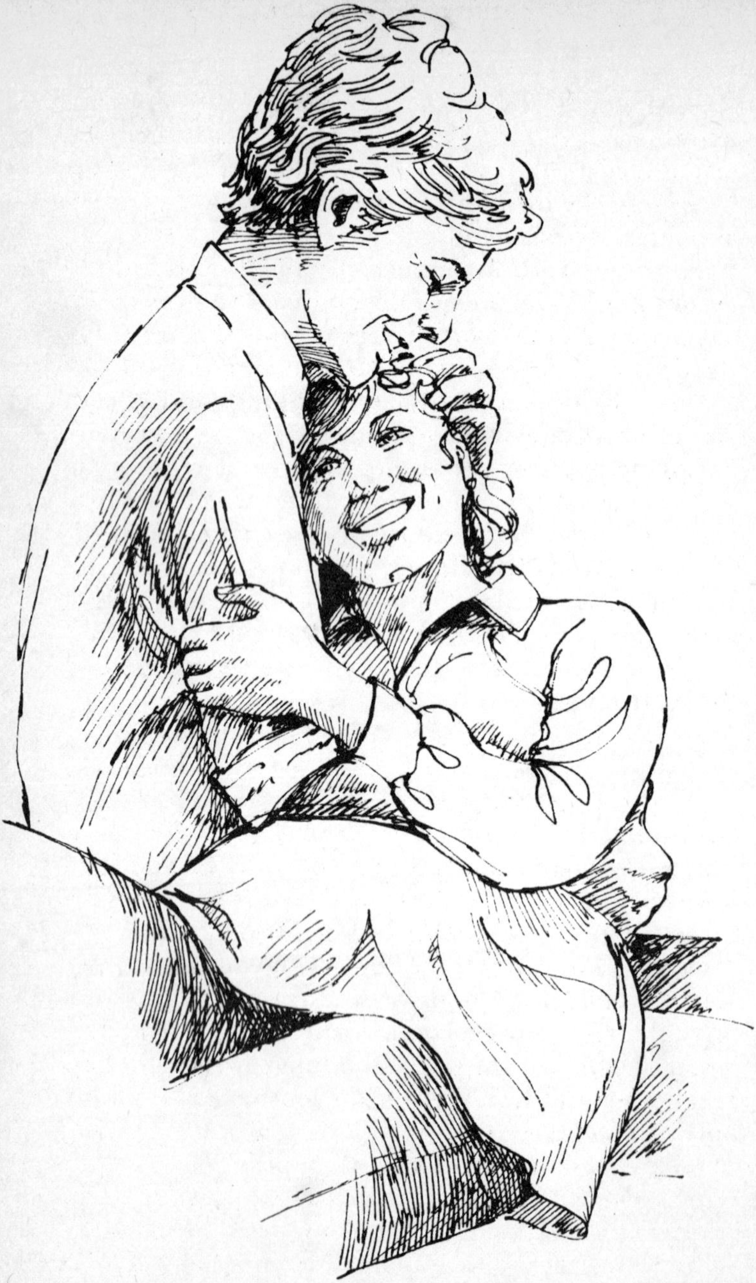

Rest and pray.

rest, and this will so rest your body that you may peacefully sleep for a while and wake refreshed and renewed.

Later in this book you can read about the art of relaxation which will be such a help to both you and your partner during pregnancy and labour and in the months ahead. Anxiety can make you feel even more weary, so try to talk over your thoughts and feelings together, or with your midwife or doctor.

> Have no anxiety about anything, but in everything by prayer and supplication with thanksgiving let your requests be made known to God. And the peace of God, which passes all understanding, will keep your hearts and your minds in Christ Jesus (Philippians 4:6-7 Revised Standard Version).

3. Exercise

Often people who are expecting a baby feel they shouldn't continue with their favourite sport or exercise, but providing you are fit and well exercise is good for you, and helps you to remain supple. A friend of mine played squash and did bell ringing throughout her pregnancy. Another used to come to antenatal classes on her bike. If the sport is very strenuous, it would be wise to ask your doctor if he considers you should continue, and should you have any dizziness or bleeding from the vagina, you should stop all exercise until you have seen your doctor and been advised by him. Remember when lifting anything, or bending down, to make your legs bend and take the weight, or you could strain your back.

Caring for your baby

1. Lovemaking

Some couples wonder if they will harm the baby when they make love. Lovemaking is the natural and wonderful way to express care and love for each other, in which the baby shares. The baby is all tucked up safely and intercourse cannot harm him. The mucus plug in the cervix and the bag of waters in the uterus act as total protectors. Only if you are naturally ready to give birth can intercourse influence the soft, ripe cervix, and labour may begin (and what a lovely way to start labour!). Intercourse will have no harmful effect. If you have had any bleeding from the vagina, or 'spotting', in early pregnancy, you should avoid intercourse at that time in each month when you would usually have had your period, and you would be wise to consult your doctor.

2. Drugs

I have already mentioned how important it is to avoid taking all drugs, unless prescribed by your doctor, during your pregnancy. When you consider the incredibly intricate development of your baby, especially in those early days and weeks of pregnancy, you will realize how vital it is to protect your baby from any substance which could be harmful. Drugs taken by you may be toxic for your baby, especially as the baby's liver and kidneys are too immature to break down toxic substances. Obviously should you need certain drugs prescribed by your doctor, to maintain your health, then it is a matter of weighing up the risks. Some drugs have not been researched sufficiently for doctors to know the risk to the developing baby; other drugs have been taken apparently safely by pregnant mums over many years. You need to discuss this with your doctor. The vital thing is not to take 'over the counter' drugs but only prescribed drugs, from a doctor who knows you are pregnant (this is another good reason for early confirmation of your pregnancy).

Don't forget that nicotine and alcohol are also drugs. Both should be avoided. The occasional glass of wine or sherry seems harmless enough, but some women cannot break down the alcohol in their bodies, so it passes through the placenta into the baby's bloodstream. The effect on the baby is not fully known, but it seems to be an unnecessary risk. However, the dangers of smoking *are* known. Nicotine passes through the placenta to the baby whether you inhale or not. The nicotine has a direct effect on the placenta, causing the blood vessels to constrict so less food and oxygen get to Baby. The baby's heartbeat increases. The result is that his growth is affected and you may give birth to an underweight baby. Also the chances of having a miscarriage and other serious problems increase. If you do smoke, make it an urgent matter and do everything in your power to stop. You can choose whether you smoke or not. Your baby doesn't have that choice!

3. German measles

Most women have either had this very mild disease, or have been safely vaccinated against it. However, if you have not had it or been vaccinated and you contract the disease during early pregnancy, there is a high chance the baby will be damaged in some way. If you think you have had the disease, or been in contact with it, see your doctor immediately.

Other vaccinations given before travelling abroad are not recommended during the first four months of pregnancy, and the smallpox vaccination should be avoided throughout the pregnancy.

4. X-rays

X-rays can affect the development of the baby. Should you need X-rays for a diagnosis, have only the minimum needed and consult your doctor as there is a risk to your baby which needs to be weighed against the advantages of the X-ray for your own health.

Hospital tests during pregnancy

There are some tests you may be offered during your pregnancy which I will briefly describe here. Should you have any of these tests, do ask the doctors all about the reasons for and results of the tests. In this way you are not made anxious and can fully understand the situation.

1. Scan or ultrasound

This is a method of gaining a picture of the baby in the uterus by bouncing very high frequency sound-waves off solid parts of the baby. This is done by passing a transducer over your oiled abdomen (it is quite painless), which then transmits this information onto a screen which you can see. It may be difficult to understand the picture you see, although sometimes the baby is clearly visible. A scan may be done to assess the baby's development, to see in which position he is lying, or even to assess the position and condition of the placenta. If the placenta is very low in the uterus, there is a danger it could bleed as the baby is born. Because of this risk you would be offered a Caesarean section. Ultrasound is believed to be far safer than X-rays.

2. Amniocentesis

This simply means removing a small amount of the fluid which surrounds the baby in the uterus so that it may be analysed. It is possible to detect some abnormalities such as mongolism or spina bifida. It is performed by passing a hollow needle through the abdomen wall under local anaesthetic, into the uterus and withdrawing some of the fluid. There is a small chance of this procedure causing a miscarriage, so a careful decision needs to be made by you both, with your doctor, weighing up the benefits and the risks for your baby.

3. AFP screening

AFP is short for Alpha-feto-protein which is a substance normally secreted by the developing embryo. A simple blood test before the eighteenth week is taken to check the AFP level. When AFP levels are unusually high it sometimes means that there may be some type of abnormality such as spina bifida.

4. Fetoscopy

This is a method of actually taking a picture of the baby inside the uterus so as to detect any abnormalities. A small incision is made under local anaesthetic through the abdominal wall and into the uterus. A fine tube with a light and lens is introduced. The whole procedure is done under a scan so as not to damage the baby.

Some pregnancy problems

Many mothers sail through pregnancy feeling not only very fit, but healthy and happy. Having said that, it is only fair to mention some problems that you may come up against. Several of these problems are as a result of the hormonal changes which occur. The hormones of pregnancy make your body ready for birth, so ligaments are softened and blood vessels are carrying extra blood. Your veins are not quite as efficient as usual and you may develop varicose veins in your legs or vagina. You will need to sit more with your feet up and do some pelvic rocking to encourage good circulation. Constipation may be a problem, in which case try adding bran to your cereals and eat plenty of high-fibre foods.

Backache and pain in the groin are fairly common problems. Are you balanced well as you walk or are you tilting backwards with a hollow in your lower back? Ask your partner to help you with your balance. Pelvic rocking can be very soothing and is good to do anyway. The uterus with all its weight causes some degree of congestion and pressure in the lower pelvic area which can cause pain in the groin. You will need to sit and rest more, avoid standing and also do more exercise between your rests to aid circulation.

Cramp, which is very painful, can occur in the calf muscles—often at night. It may mean you are not getting enough calcium, in which case you should see your doctor. Sometimes eating something salty last thing at night helps. Should you get cramp, try stretching out the affected muscle by standing on the leg with the cramp and leaning slightly forward, or ask your husband to stretch your foot up, while pressing firmly on your knee. Stay like that until the muscle spasm has passed, then gently massage it. Try not to curl your toes under as this can start cramp.

The rising uterus squashes the stomach a little, leaving less room for heavy meals. The pregnancy hormones relax muscles, and this includes the muscle which keeps the acid stomach juices from leaking back into the gullet, or oesophagus. This causes an uncomfortable burning sensation, known as 'heartburn'. Try taking light snacks rather than heavy meals, and prop yourself up well with pillows in bed so that gravity helps the juices to stay in the stomach. If heartburn becomes a serious problem see your doctor, who may prescribe some mild form of antacid.

These problems are common and you can usually learn to cope with them at home. Pregnancy is not an illness and at no time should you feel ill. If you do then go to your doctor; he can check your blood pressure, make sure you are not anaemic, or have too much sugar in your blood. Should you at any time during your pregnancy develop very severe headaches, go to your doctor immediately, as it may mean your blood pressure has gone up too far. Likewise, should you get any bleeding from the vagina see your doctor without delay.

Caring together

You have seen how you can care for one another and for your baby during pregnancy. It really is a time when your love overflows from one to the other and back again. When we learn to love ourselves, that love embraces others. We first learn about love by the love our mothers show us by the light of their countenance, through their eyes, their tender smile for us. I believe that love can start in pregnancy.

Some people scorn the need to love themselves even though it is Christ's command to us to 'love your neighbour as yourself'. People get all tied up with religious guilt, self-negation—a sort of martyrdom which just isn't what Jesus taught and doesn't reflect the truth about our experiences in life.

We cannot give love if we have not first received it. We receive it by the grace of our Lord Jesus Christ, shown to us in our mothers' love, by a loved one, or sometimes simply by him who loves us so completely. He loves us as we are, in us, by us, because of us and in spite of us. We are loved people. We love and value ourselves knowing we are his children, made in his image. We need that comfort, that understanding, that love; for then having received we can give, having been pardoned we can forgive, having received the gift of life we may invest it for him and discover eternal life. We need a 'theology of the self'. The church so often preaches heroic self-negation instead of non-heroic self-affirmation! Pregnancy is a time of self-affirmation, of self-awareness, of wholeness.

'All things come from you, and of thine own do we give you.'

Father we bring before you
All that this pregnancy entails.
Our excitement, our anxieties,
Our troubles and our joys.
Accept our frailty, and know that
We put our trust in you.
The days are long, and tiredness
And tears blend with rest and praise.
Together we seek to do your will,
Together we grow in love.
We go on our way rejoicing.
Thanks be to God. Amen.

CHAPTER FOUR

Guiding Thy Steps

How your baby is born
Relaxation for life
Relaxation technique
Breathing for labour
Positions for labour
Coping with pain
Relating to hospital staff
Prayer

How your baby is born

YOU HAVE JOURNEYED on through nine long months of pregnancy. You may be impatient now to actually give birth. I love that word, to 'give' birth, because it is in giving your body, mind and spirit over to the great birth experience that you will receive that unspeakable gift from God, your new baby. Your body is a superb machine, beautifully designed and now fully prepared to give birth. All you need to do is to allow, to give, and to 'go with' the natural feelings and forces you experience. Birth is a miracle, a great mystery of God, and it is both thrilling and a little awe inspiring to be at the centre of that mystery. The forces of God are immense and unrelenting as your body first prepares for the baby's journey through the birth canal, and then as it helps to ease and guide him out into the world.

It will help you greatly if you have a clear picture of what is actually happening to you and your baby during labour. The baby's head usually sinks deep down into the pelvis sometime during the last four weeks of pregnancy. This means the head is deeply engaged in the pelvis and pressing on the cervix. Just occasionally, the baby decides to sit the other way round with its head high up under your ribs and its bottom down in the pelvis. This is called a 'breech' position or presentation, and your doctor will need to decide whether to let you go ahead with a normal vaginal delivery, or whether a Caesarean birth might be safer for you and your baby.

With the birth imminent, the cervix which has become soft and ripe for labour gently begins to shorten and thin as bands of muscle through the uterus tighten up and relax, then tighten up (or contract) again. You may have noticed this tightening up during the latter part of pregnancy. These are practice contractions called 'Braxton Hicks', and may have given you a good idea of how contractions come and go at the beginning of your labour. Now the cervix will be thinned, or 'effaced', and will be drawn up into the lower section of the uterus. During the past nine months there has been a plug of mucus blocking the canal which runs through the cervix to help protect the baby. With the movement of the cervix this plug of mucus falls away through the vagina. This is called a 'show'. You may notice it as a thick, jelly-like substance which is often slightly blood stained. As the contractions gain in strength and regularity, the canal in the cervix starts to open or dilate. The whole of the first stage of your labour is simply the dilating of the cervix. The pressure of the baby's head on the dilating cervix helps it to dilate more quickly and easily, and you will read in the following chapter how keeping upright helps this pressure to be maintained.

It may take up to twelve hours, or more, for the muscles of the uterus to pull the cervix open by the ever-increasing contractions. The baby is wrapped in a bag of water sealed in by a membrane. With the dilatation of the cervix, the bag bursts at some stage and some of the fluid drains out. Occasionally this happens at the very start of labour. Eventually the cervix becomes fully dilated and this is the stage called transition because it is a transition from the first to the second stage of labour. Once the cervix is fully dilated to 10cm, then the baby is free to begin his journey down through the birth canal. At this time the contractions, which have become very strong and close together, change in their nature as the uterus now presses and eases the baby down the birth passage and out into the world. These contractions give your body a strong desire to help to ease, push and guide the baby out.

As the baby gets lower, so your vagina will ease and stretch out around him—the muscles are very elastic. With each contraction the baby's head moves forward, then slips back a little, then forward a little more, until the head can be seen in the vagina. The pelvic floor, or perineum, bulges and the skin at the vaginal outlet slips back over the baby's head. Once the head is born, it turns sideways to be in line with the shoulders. With the next contraction, the shoulders are born and your baby's body quickly and gently slithers out with a gush of water!

While you love and cherish your little babe, your body is finishing the birth. The placenta, which has been the baby's life support, now peels off the inside lining of the uterus as it finally shrinks down. The placenta, umbilical cord and membranes now flop down into the vagina and are expelled with another small contraction. The umbilical cord may be clamped and cut now as the placenta is no longer needed, and Baby is using his lungs and breathing by himself. The delivery of the placenta is called the third stage of labour.

The whole labour and birth experience may be thrilling, dramatic and very tiring. It will be a time of strong physical and emotional feelings. Some of these feelings may be painful, some overwhelming, some enjoyable. You can explore these feelings more in the next chapter and learn how to help each other during labour: relaxation with special breathing patterns can be a great help. It is also very valuable to have thought about pain and how your mind and body may adapt and cope with it if experienced.

Relaxation for life

Relaxation can be so valuable, not just during labour but during our entire lives. Think of the wasted energy we burn up by being physically and mentally tense. Next time you're late for an appointment, or someone is critically watching you in the kitchen, or you're at a social function with your boss, pause for a while and notice how tense you may have become. Be aware of the pressure of thought, how your mind is rushing. Notice how your arms and legs, your neck and back feel almost stiff. Feel your tense fingers, your anxious face, your taut muscles. Your whole body is using up far more energy than it need. That is energy wasted—it could be used far more creatively. Using up energy means you soon become tired and require rest, but you cannot even rest properly if you're tense. Some people are so tense they are wearing their bodies down, and eventually suffer from one of the stress-related diseases such as stomach ulcers, heart strain or high blood pressure. It is abuse of our bodies, and I'm quite sure God doesn't mean us to live like that.

Take a look at your life now, before you get into a vicious cycle of work, tension, poor rest, etc. and learn to keep calm, confident and relaxed. The meditation at the end of this chapter is a beautiful, quiet reflection on peace, and our ability to rest and relax and to hear the still small voice of calm. This verse in particular is so right for relaxation:

> Drop thy still dews of quietness,
> Till all our strivings cease;
> Take from our souls the strain and stress,
> And let our ordered lives confess
> The beauty of thy peace.
>
> *Whittier*

If only our lives could be like that. But how do we relax? First, relaxation is not lying down in a darkened room, and feeling like a wet fish on a fish slab! Relaxation is rather a way of resting, so that we use only essential energy, while being aware of our body, and in tune with its needs and responses. Think of a violinist playing the violin. He adjusts his poise, his balance, his strength and his bow to get the tone. He feels the intensity or softness of the note, he is in tune with the music's emotional feel, he is in time with the orchestra, he knows instinctively when to be creatively tense and when to be relaxed so as to find the perfect harmony. You need to discover something like that sensitivity and be as relaxed as that to discover the harmony in life, or to be in tune with your body through labour and to hear that 'still voice of calm'.

Relaxation is an art that needs to be learned and practised. Once you know and remember how your body feels when it is relaxed you have the key to success. You can practise the following relaxation technique to become aware of relaxation. Once you have the right feel in your body, you can use a very quick method, a wave of relaxation, which should achieve the same simply as you breathe out—ideal in labour

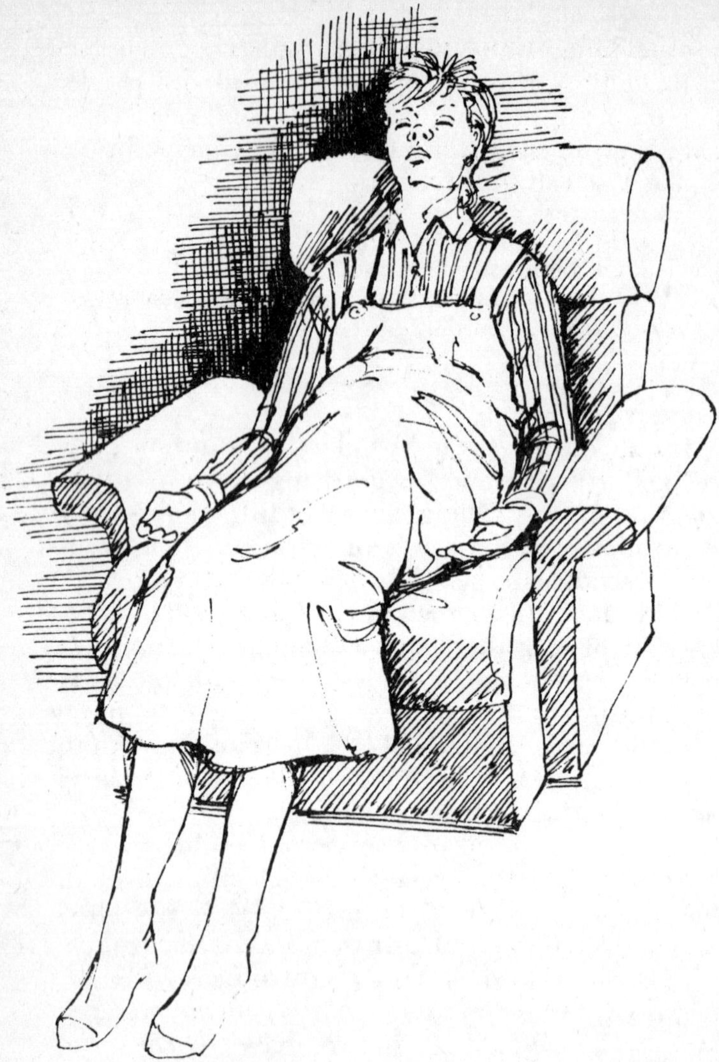

There are just four words to remember:
smile, shoulders, soft, still.

or in stressful situations in everyday life. You can try this method with your partner.

Relaxation technique

Try to bring to your time of relaxation all that is good and positive in your life. Believe in your own value as a person. Follow these simple instructions:

1. Smile as you take a slow deep breath in, then sigh it all out. Leave your lips slightly parted as you breathe gently and naturally.

2. Close your eyes and feel a smoothness spread out wide between your eyes, up through your hair, and down to the back of your neck, and rest.

3. Pull your shoulders down towards your feet. Stop, and now turn the palms of your hands uppermost.

4. Stretch out your fingers, long and hard. Now stop, and feel a plump softness flow through your hands and fingers.

5. Gently press your pelvis down into the cushions. Stop, and feel a softness flow over your abdomen and round to the small of your back. Feel your weight completely supported by the cushions.

6. Straighten your legs, feet slightly apart. Pull your feet and toes up towards your face. Now stop, and allow your legs to sink heavily into the floor, and be still.

7. Lean on love. Know that you are loved, lovable and lovely. Quietly give thanks to God.

8. Slowly, in your own time, move your fingers, hands and arms. Gently move your toes, feet and legs. Open your eyes, stretch, and gradually come back to your

usual activity.

Once you have practised this relaxation several times and you have experienced some good relaxation, you will become accustomed to the feeling of your body once the muscles are no longer tense. It is that awareness of relaxation which is so important. You may now like to try a far quicker method of relaxing which is basically the same. It should enable you to relax completely as you sigh out that first breath.

There are just four words to remember:

Smile
Shoulders
Soft
Still

Say them slowly over to yourself.

As you say 'smile' you will relax your face, mouth, head and neck. As you say 'shoulder' you will relax your shoulders, arms and hands and fingers. As you say 'soft' you will relax your abdomen, back and pelvis. As you say 'still' you will relax your thighs, calf muscles, feet and toes.

Eventually you may become so good at relaxing that you only need to repeat the first word 'smile' to be able to set off the relaxation wave through all parts of your body. Try it at various times of the day, in different situations, and become an expert in the art of relaxation. Eventually you may be able to meet tension with relaxation, literally, as you breathe out. Think of the advantage to you as you sit in the car, or do the ironing, or breastfeed your baby. Try it in church, in the supermarket, or when you next have a disagreement with your partner! It is a flowing out feeling, outwards towards life and love, a meeting with pain and tension, a befriending of stress and a gathering of peace. It is a giving of your true inner self into the hands of God. Smile and enjoy him.

Breathing for labour

It seems strange to have to think of telling anyone how to breathe. Breathing is a natural process in which your body takes in the amount of oxygen needed for the task in hand. If you run for a bus you will naturally increase your breathing. If you are relaxing well your breathing will be calm and steady. The problem only arises when you are stressed. Think what happens to your breathing when you stub your toe painfully, or hammer your thumb instead of a nail! The result may be breath-holding, or sharp erratic breaths while you tense up and rub the injured part.

While you are in labour the uterus is working extremely hard. There may be an immense tightening and gripping feeling over your abdomen during a contraction. There may be a little or a lot of pain. Your breathing will need to change in response to the work, pressure or pain you are feeling. If you learn a pattern of breathing, you will have a guideline in your mind which you can use during a contraction. This will lead you to calm, controlled breathing. You won't become short of oxygen, nor will your baby, and you won't be tempted to overbreathe and become panicky.

To begin with, work together and help each other to discover these different types of breathing:

1. Start by placing your hands just below waist level, each side of your tummy. Breathe in slowly and deeply to the level of your hands, then sigh it all out. This can be your 'greeting' breath for each new contraction. It will give you and your baby plenty of

oxygen in preparation for the hard work of the contraction to come. You can also combine this greeting breath with your code for relaxation, and have a wave of relaxation as you breathe out. Don't forget to smile!

2. Now place your hands either side of your chest wall, under your arms. Breathe in gently to the level of your hands. In, out, pause, in, out, pause. This breathing is steady and rhythmical. Find the pace that is comfortable for you. This is useful as the contraction becomes stronger because the lighter breathing lifts pressure off your diaphragm from the top of your uterus.

3. Next place your hands over your shoulders with fingers cupped over towards your back. Now breathe very very lightly, concentrating on the out-breath—the in-breath will take care of itself. Think that you are gently flapping a piece of tissue paper, or lifting a tiny feather on the palm of your hand. Find your own rhythm. This is very useful when the contraction becomes extremely strong. You can think of riding up over the crest of the wave of the contraction with this very light breathing while your body relaxes around your uterus, which is then free to work hard and well.

If at any time you feel dizzy, or you develop tingly fingers, then you are overbreathing. Simply breathe in and out of cupped hands quite sharply for two or three breaths, and this should put you right.

4. There may come a time in the transition stage when your body feels it wants to push with the contraction, but the midwife may ask you not to push yet until she is sure your cervix is fully dilated. It is hard to control the urge to push, but if you breathe lightly and distinctly in a pattern of 'who-who-ha-ha' pause,

'who-who-ha-ha' pause, this should help you to overcome the pushing urge until you are free to go ahead.

5. Once you are in the second stage and the midwife says you may now push with each contraction, your breathing will naturally change, but it is tempting to take a deep breath in and hold it and push, and hold it further until you (and your baby) go blue in the face! This will soon exhaust you and tire your baby. You may also find yourself pushing up through your face rather than downwards as you open up and give birth. The word 'push' is not really very helpful. Better to think of 'leaning' on the contraction as you bear down. Take one or two fairly deep breaths in and out as the contraction starts. When you feel the urge to bear down, breathe in, hold your breath while you lean on the contraction. Then let the breath go when it feels natural to do so. Quickly breathe in and out again once or twice, hold the breath, and lean on it again, feeling the strength of the contraction to guide your breathing. Next, as the urge to bear down fades, let your breath go, take a deep breath in and out, along with a ripple of relaxation, and smile. You can read more about the different types of contractions and how to cope with them in the next chapter.

Relaxation with breathing for labour is not just a technique to learn. It is part of your co-operation with your labour. It can be a breathing in of God's goodness, oxygen to sustain you and your baby, and his Spirit of care and comfort which infuses your baby as you labour with him.

Try putting the breathing levels together now as if you are having a contraction. As the contraction begins relax, take a deep greeting breath in, and let it go, and relax again. As the contraction gains in strength, lighten your breathing up to mid-chest, steady and rhythmical. Now the contraction is really very strong, so use your shoulder breathing with its quick, very light breathing—like the flapping of butterfly wings. As the contraction lessens, drop the breathing down to mid-chest for a while, then when you feel the contraction fade away, take a deep resting breath, in and out, as you relax and smile. Remember it is essential to combine your breathing with the relaxation you have learned.

Positions for labour

A good position is yet another tool that will help you through labour. Women used to adopt whatever position they were most comfortable in, until a gentleman in France decided women should lie on their backs to produce babies! Unfortunately it was a queen of France who was so persuaded, and the fashion of lying down in childbirth became popular. It is only in recent years that people have realized that lying down causes women to have longer, more painful labours. More pain led to more drugs, more exhaustion and more complicated deliveries. However, you can really thank God that things have changed. It is now known, and accepted, that staying upright in the first stage of labour helps gravity to press the baby's head onto the dilating cervix, resulting in quicker and more even dilatation. The uterus can contract down onto the baby, helping to push him down in the second stage through the birth canal. The vagina is at right angles to the uterus, so the baby has a bend to negotiate. If you are flat on your back you have to push the baby up against gravity!

In the first stage, stay upright for as long as possible, walking around carrying out your normal housework. You may like to lean against a wall for a contraction, or lean onto a table, or lean against your husband with your arms around his neck. When the contractions become stronger try various positions. An excellent position is to sit back to front astride an upright chair with a cushion on the top on which to rest your head and arms. You can sit and watch television like that while you enjoy your labour. The pelvis is at just the right angle to help you most. Kneeling up against a low settee is another very good position, with a pillow under your knees and another over your heels to sit back on if you wish. Try different positions, especially during a long labour. Some labours may cause backache in which case it would be good to get onto all fours for some contractions as it brings the baby's weight off your back. You may feel best sitting upright with plenty of cushions. At any time throughout labour it is helpful and often comforting to do pelvic rocking. The movement will add stimulation to the dilating cervix. It will help the baby's head to descend in second stage and negotiate the bend in the birth canal.

During the second stage, it is more difficult to move as you feel very heavy. If you've discussed positions early on with your midwife, she will know how to help you change positions. Any of the positions of first stage are possible and helpful now. You might like to squat to have your baby, but this is best if you are supported. You can buy a little plastic toddler step (you'll need it later on anyway) and this is ideal for sitting on in second stage. It has a slight hollow in front and is just the right height. A rolled up towel on the top will make it more comfortable. A full, unsupported squat can cause too much strain on the tissues of the perineum. If you want to squat, have one person each side of you fully supporting your weight.

Changing position, along with relaxation and breathing, is yet another way in which you can help yourself through labour. Being in tune with your body, listening to its needs, and being aware of its feelings or language, will help you enormously to adapt to the natural most beneficial breathing, resting, and positions for you and your baby.

Nobody can do it as well as you can!

Coping with pain

How do you cope with pain? Think back to a painful experience. Did you pretend it was not there? Did you shout or scream? Were you frightfully 'stiff upper lip'? Did you grin and bear it? It is helpful to think how you and your family cope with pain, how you've been brought up to deal with pain, and to try to understand why you react as you do.

Some fear over pain is not only about the actual pain, but what your reaction to the pain will be. You may fear you will lose control of yourself, or cry out, or somehow look silly and let yourself down. But who are you afraid of upsetting? God doesn't mind if you shout or get angry—he understands. Your partner will be so involved, he'll understand too. There *is* a dignity in childbirth, no matter how undignified your physical position! If you should feel you will lose control, trust in the skill of the midwives, and let go in the arms of God.

The pain of childbirth is a fulfilling pain. There is no other pain like it. It is creative pain, it may be pleasurable pain, and it is very soon forgotten as you are caught up in the joy of the birth of your baby. I've experienced three very different births myself, so I understand something of the pain of childbirth. The first delivery was a long and highly technical hospital experience. The second, a difficult home delivery, and the third was a fabulous Domino delivery—very hard work, but exciting and beautiful. If you can go with the pain, and not tense up against it, if you can greet it as a further step towards seeing and holding your baby, if you accept it as part of the wonder and mystery of birth, you will have no fear. Some women experience only immense pressure, some have discomfort, some have pain. For some, the first stage is painful, and the second stage exhilarating. Others find the first stage easy and enjoyable, and yet find pain in the actual birth. No one knows how it will be for you, but it's not an exam you're taking, there's no pass or fail—you are unique, your labour is unique, just as your baby is unique. You can help yourself by using relaxation, special breathing and by changing your position. Should you need more help, the hospital may offer you gas and air, drugs or anaesthesia —which you can learn more about later in this book. It is important to know that there is help for you if you feel a lot of pain, but it is equally helpful to know that pain in childbirth is indescribably different, and can be a wonderful and very pleasurable experience as you give your body over to the delivery of your child.

God doesn't send you pain to punish you for being bad, nor does he stand callously by. There is a story of a very religious man who, when his village was threatened with a flood, insisted God would save him. The waters reached the first floor of his house and villagers sent a boat to rescue him, but he refused saying, 'God will save me.' The waters reached the roof tops and the villagers sent a helicopter. 'No,' said the man, 'God will save me.' The man drowned and went to heaven. He went to see God and said, 'Now look here, I'm very angry with you for not rescuing me from the flood!' God quietly said to him, 'Oh, but I did send you a boat and a helicopter.'

So in labour, God has given us bodies perfectly designed to give birth; the ability to use relaxation, breathing and change of position. He also gives skilled midwives, drugs, anaesthetics and skilled surgeons should they be necessary. If labour is hard for you, give thanks that you have so much help, and accept it all as being part of the maturing process which is called motherhood!

Relating to hospital staff

Midwives and doctors are usually very pleasant people who want you to enjoy your birth experience, and who will help you all they can. The midwife/mother/father relationship is intimate and precious, and it is largely up to you to give all you can to make it a success. Chat to your midwife as a friend. Get to know her as a person. If you are going into hospital, begin this good relationship as soon as you arrive. Ask the midwife her name, thank her for all she does for you, and above all talk to her as an adult. It is so easy when things are being done for you by professional people to fall into the trap of suddenly feeling like a young child being looked after by an all-powerful mother!

Talk to your midwife as early as you can about the sort of labour you are hoping for. Talk to her about positions and breathing so that she understands how she can help you most. Do ask intelligent questions. 'Is everything all right?' will probably be answered with a 'yes, dear', but to ask how dilated the cervix is, or what is the position of the baby's head, should impress and interest your midwife, and you'll soon be drawn together as *three* people doing all they can to help each other.

If you are worried about your labour, or if you have strong feelings about the type of labour you hope for, it would be wise to write a letter to your consultant before you go into labour, expressing your hopes. However, do remember that no one knows how your labour is going to go, so try to remain flexible in your attitude. You, or your baby, may need help. I feel the word 'intervention' conjures up a picture of unnecessary interference. That is something to avoid, but real help, aid, may be vital for you or your baby. A 'natural' delivery, free from all technical aid or drugs, is far more likely if you can accept that help is there for you if you need it, but you cannot insist on a natural delivery. Baby may get too tired, or get into a difficult position. Co-operating with modern medicine may be your way of letting God help you to have a healthy baby. If, on the other hand, you feel there is unnecessary technology, and you are coping well and labour is progressing, then simply be very pleasant but very firm with the midwives, and insist that while everything is all right you don't wish for any unnecessary intervention.

You are now ready to share the birthday of your child. You know what is happening to your body and your baby. You have learned how to relax and rest, how to breathe through contractions, and you know about the importance of finding a suitable position. While you relate happily to the midwives and medical staff, you can feel confident not only in their skill but also in the ability of your body, so perfectly designed for this work of labour, and you can be confident in the continuing care of your heavenly Father. As you labour together—giving, sharing, helping, loving—know that the kingdom of heaven is between you in your love for each other, for your babe, and in your love for God and his love for you. He is there for you. His love for you is superabundant. He suffers with you and rejoices with you. He's that kind of God.

Lord Jesus Christ, we come before you
In simple trust, knowing that you
Love us and want only good for us.
Guide us now as we prepare
For the birth of this babe.
Help us to learn to rest in your arms,
To sleep in your peace,
And to wake refreshed and renewed
In the light of your countenance.
Grant us freedom from fear,
Fulfilment in birth,
And delight in your goodness. Amen.

CHAPTER FIVE

Truth in Its Beauty

Prelude to labour
Labour begins
Giving birth
God's gift to you
Your gift to him
Prayer

A WOMAN IN labour is beautiful. Her skin is moist and flushed, her eyes are shining, her hair tangled. It is a time of truth, no pretence, no airs and graces, but simply a natural working to bring about the birth of a child. As labour progresses, the mother withdraws into her own emotional, spiritual and physical world. She may say little. She knows instinctively how to move for her own comfort and how also to help the baby's position. Many of the suitable positions for birth are like positions of prayer—again a time of withdrawal. Helpers at this time need to allow the natural responses of the mother to take place. It is rather a matter of tenderness, not technique. As the time of birth approaches, there needs to be calm and quiet, gentle encouragement and physical support. There should be no hurry. As the baby's head is born the mother may naturally cry out—a mixture of pain, pleasure, release and joy. As she cuddles and suckles the baby she is complete. She is fulfilled. A new family is born.

Prelude to labour

In the days before labour the cervix softens and becomes 'ripe'. It is normal to go into labour anytime between two weeks before or two weeks after your expected date of delivery. Should labour start before the thirty-eighth week of pregnancy you should telephone the hospital. The Braxton Hicks contractions you may have felt in the past weeks may become stronger, and these contractions will gently thin out and draw up the soft cervix into the lower section of the uterus, ready for labour to dilate the cervix. During these last days of your pregnancy you may feel impatient or even irritable. You may long to start labour, or you may cherish these last days when you and your baby are still one being. You may feel overactive and want to decorate or clean the house or finish the gardening! It's best if you keep active, but don't exhaust yourself as you will need all your energy for the birth day.

Immediately before labour you may feel a fullness, almost a period pain, low down in your pelvis, or perhaps a similar pain deep in your back. Some mums have diarrhoea just before labour starts, others just know they feel strange, and inexplicably feel that today is the day! It is good to share all these feelings with your partner so that he is involved right from the start. This is his baby and his labour as well as yours, and it is exciting to share the secret that labour is very near, and to prayerfully await its onset.

Labour begins

Each labour has its own unique way of beginning, but you may find that one of three things happens:

1. Show

You may discover that you have had a show, and that the mucus plug in the cervix has fallen away because the cervix has thinned out or even begun to dilate. This is very exciting, and it may be that you will now go into labour. However, it is not uncommon to have a show several days or even a week or two before labour. Take it as an encouraging sign that things may be starting to happen, and wait and see.

2. Waters

The bag of waters which has enveloped your baby may burst as the cervix moves. Occasionally the waters go with a great gush, but there is more likely to be a slow trickle. You will need to wear a pad, and a plastic sheet under your bed linen is a wise precaution.

If the waters go with a gush you should telephone the hospital immediately. They may send an ambulance to take you safely into hospital where the hospital staff will be able to check that the baby's umbilical cord has not been washed down into the vagina with the gush of waters. If you are only losing a trickle of water, and providing you are comfortable, you can continue to stay active at home for a few more hours, but this should not exceed twelve hours as there could be a risk of infection in the uterus, so telephone the hospital and seek their advice.

3. Contractions

It may be that the mild Braxton Hicks contractions of the past few days become far stronger, and may also become regular. When labour becomes established you can expect regular contractions, say, every ten minutes or a little less. These contractions will gradually increase in strength. Sometimes a show appears with regular contractions, or the waters might break —possibly causing contractions to get stronger and closer together. Once you realize that the contractions are regular, it is a good idea to make a note of exactly when they are coming, and how long they are lasting. In this way you can keep an accurate record of what is happening through your labour and this will help you and the hospital staff.

The beginning of labour can be a very exciting time. You've both waited a long time for this, now there's no turning back! It can also make you anxious. You are embarking on a journey which will culminate in the birth of your child, but no one knows what sort of journey it will be. This is an intimate time, a time of anticipation which you can share together.

One couple I taught had a visit from Mum while they were in the early first stage of labour. They felt strongly that this was their special time, their secret, and throughout this fairly brief and happy visit they didn't tell her about it! That's fine, it is a very special time, one to be savoured and treasured as you work together in labour. It can also be a time of smiles, and tears, cuddles and kisses. As the contractions become more intense, you will need to greet them with your breathing and relaxation, and find different comfortable positions. Many couples go for a walk during early labour. One of my NCT class went to have her hair done, and breathed quietly through contractions without the hairdresser realizing she was in labour!

If labour is not progressing too quickly, it would be good to have a very nutritious meal so as to boost your energy reserves. You may have a long way to go, perhaps a whole day and night. If you really feel you couldn't face a meal, it may mean you are more advanced than you think, so suck some glucose sweets or tablets, or have a spoonful of honey with a drink.

You may wonder when to go into hospital, and as every labour is different it is not easy to advise you. However, once fairly strong contractions are coming every five minutes, then it would be wise to telephone the hospital, and be prepared to go in if that is their advice. It is good to get to hospital before the enormous contractions, which herald the end of first stage, occur as this would not only be very uncomfortable for you, but it would give you no time to get to know the hospital staff. As you journey to the hospital, it may be most comfortable to sit on the back seat of the car so you can lean over the top of the front seat during contractions. Take a towel with you in case your waters break, and a plastic bag in case you're sick! Breathe gently through contractions, use your relaxation as far as possible, and smile.

Here are some suggestions of what to take with you into hospital. It is helpful to have three small bags instead of one large one. One bag for labour, one for your needs after labour, and one with Baby's clothes and shawl, etc.

1. Small natural sponge—for bathing face, wetting lips
2. Hot and cold picnic packs—for comfort
3. Ice cubes in thermos—to suck
4. Mister plant spray—for cooling down
5. Woolly socks or leg warmers—for warmth
6. Lip salve or vaseline—for dry lips
7. Cream or talc—for massage
8. Front opening nightdresses—for breast feeding
9. Glucose tablets or honey—for energy
10. Food, sandwiches, chocolate—for hungry Dad
11. Music on tape, books, playing cards—for a long

labour

12. Extra cushions in the car—hospital may not have enough
13. Favourite picture with Blutak—to concentrate, meditate on
14. At least three nursing bras—for comfort and support
15. Note pad and pencil—for labour log
16. Plenty of change—for telephone calls
17. Bran—to prevent constipation after birth
18. Smile—for you and midwife and Baby to enjoy the birth day!

When you arrive at the hospital you will be welcomed by a midwife. She will ask you about your labour so far, and she may examine you internally to assess the dilatation of the cervix. Some midwives suggest you have a pubic shave. Research has shown that this procedure is of no actual value, and that it can cause discomfort. If you don't wish to have a shave, explain this pleasantly but firmly to the midwife.

Likewise, it may be suggested that you have an enema or suppository to clear your bowels. Again, there is no real advantage in this, unless you are very constipated. It can cause discomfort to have an enema when contractions are strong. Explain politely and firmly if you don't wish to have an enema. Dads can make excellent mediators here! Better still would be to have discussed all this and your hopes for labour in advance with the hospital staff, and to have your requests written down in your notes in the form of a pleasant, flexible letter to the consultant.

You may be offered a bath, and this is a lovely way to relax and fill in time, but make sure you and your partner stay together so he can help you through contractions. Don't forget that he may think your contractions are worse than they are—so once they're over relax, give him a smile and a kiss, and let him know you're coping beautifully. Equally, should you feel you need help, or you are anxious, talk to each other about it between contractions, and ask for help.

The midwives will want to know that the baby's heartbeat is strong and healthy. These days a monitor is used to record the baby's heartbeat along with your contraction. You can see the recording of the heartbeat on the monitor screen, and this can be very reassuring to you and the staff. A belt is fastened round your abdomen with the monitor attached. This does restrict your ability to move freely, however, so once you've been attached to the monitor for about twenty minutes, and providing all is well, do ask to come off it so you can be fully mobile again. Occasionally, if your waters have broken, the doctor may want to clip an electrode onto your baby's scalp so as to obtain a clearer recording of his heartbeat. We don't know how the baby feels about this and, again, it will make you far less mobile. If there is a problem with his welfare, then you will need to be guided by the medical team, but it would be sad to be attached to an internal foetal monitor if it wasn't absolutely necessary. Some hospitals are now equipped with portable monitors so you are free to walk around. This is obviously ideal.

Towards the end of the first stage of labour the contractions may become very strong, and you may need as much encouragement as possible. It will help greatly if your partner is able to breathe through difficult contractions with you, keeping eye-to-eye contact to help you to concentrate. At the height of a very hard contraction you may like to use some form of distraction, like tapping out your favourite tune with your fingers, or counting backwards from a hundred. Talk about this before you go into labour so you both know the plan. Your partner can help so much now by sponging your face with cold water, moistening your lips, giving you ice cubes to suck, or by firmly massaging your back, or wherever you need comfort or feel tense. He can remind you about your relaxation breathing and tell you that you're wonderful and that he loves you. You can have a short prayer together, read a psalm, or simply remind each other of God's goodness and faithfulness.

Some mothers have an obvious transition stage, while for some it goes unnoticed. You may suddenly feel that you're too tired to cope any more; you may feel very cold and shaky, or you may be sick. Sometimes women become tearful or angry. They decide they don't want this baby anyway and they want to go home! This is typical of transition. It can be a very difficult stage with contractions coming fast and furious, lasting over a minute, and coming every two minutes. You will need all the encouragement, praise and help you can get at this time. It is good to be reminded that this is probably transition (check this with your midwife), that the cervix is almost fully dilated and that soon you will be able to work with your body to ease your baby out into the world. When you feel an urge to push, which may begin as a catch in your throat, you will need to know if it is safe to push, and whether the cervix is fully dilated or not. The midwife may examine you internally. Until you have been assessed, try to overcome the urge to push by using the 'who-who-ha-ha' breathing mentioned in chapter 4. Fortunately this stage is usually brief, and it should be welcomed as it heralds the beginning of the second stage, and soon you will be holding your precious baby.

Giving birth

> The joy which a man finds in his work and which transforms the tears and sweat of it into happiness and delight—that joy is God. The wonder and curiosity which welcomes what is new and regards it not as threatening but enriching life—that wonder and curiosity is God. The confidence which leads us to abandon the shelter of our disguises and to open up the doors of our personality so that others may enter there, and both we and they be richer for the contact—that confidence is God. The vision which enables us to see the majesty of men, of all men including ourselves, piercing through the ugliness of the obscuring pathology to the beauty of the real person—that power of vision is God. The sense of belonging to the natural world, the exhilarating certainty that all things are ours whether things in Heaven or things on earth—that sense of belonging is God. The superabundance which leads us naturally and inevitably to give, not as a matter of duty nor in a spirit of patronage, but because we cannot forbear—that superabundance is God. The compelling conviction that in spite of all evidence to the contrary, in spite of all the suffering we may have to witness or undergo, the universe is on our side, and works not for our destruction but for our fulfilment—that compelling conviction is God. [H. A. Williams, *The True Wilderness* (Constable), page 117.]

This quotation from Harry Williams could have been written for the birth experience! If you seek God you can find him throughout. Giving birth is a dramatic, overwhelming, intense affair. God is in the power, the naturalness, the pain and the delight.

It can be immensely exciting when you realize you are able to work with your body to ease your baby into the world. Your whole body is taken over by a desire to expel the baby. Now is the time to change your position, perhaps sitting right up, well supported with cushions, or kneeling back on your heels, or maybe you'll feel most comfortable on all fours. Some women like to turn around to face the head of the bed and kneel, leaning forward into the pillows. Your partner can help tremendously here by supporting, steadying, or holding you with his arms around your shoulders. He can remind you to take in one or two fairly deep breaths, then hold your breath and lean on the contraction for a count of about five or six; to then let your breath go, take in two or three breaths, hold it and lean on the contraction again. You can repeat this until the urge to bear down fades.

Then there is a heaven-sent rest of perhaps three or four minutes before another contraction comes. Use this break to relax, rest and adore one another in this incredibly beautiful time. It is good to have quiet and calm, even dimmed lights if your midwife will agree. There should be as few people in the room as possible, and any onlookers who urge you to keep pushing should be pleasantly and firmly discouraged. Mothers know instinctively how to give birth, and if you are told to push more and more there is a danger you will go blue in the face and both you and baby will become short of oxygen at this vital time. Simply tuck your chin down on your chest, have soft slightly parted lips and lean on the contraction. Say yes to Baby, yes to God. Allow your body to bulge as the baby's head comes right down low in the birth outlet. Now Dad will be able to see part of the baby's head looking a little like a hamburger! It may recede between contractions, only to descend further with the next. You can put your hands down and feel your baby's head and his wet hair. As the head reaches the birth outlet, so you may have an incredible almost preposterous feeling of burning, splitting—intense pleasure mixed with pain. Let it all happen, go with it.

The midwife may ask you to pant gently as the head is born, so that you breathe your baby out gently and beautifully. There may be a pause now as the baby's rather bluish wrinkled head rotates round so it comes into line with the shoulders. The midwife may suck out the baby's mouth with a fine catheter so that it is clear for his first breath. With the next contraction, the body slithers out into the world with a gush of water! Your precious babe is born, and the sense of relief and overwhelming joy are beyond description. Baby may be placed directly onto your tummy so you can cherish and adore him as the third stage of labour takes place. If you suckle Baby at the breast immediately this will calm and reassure him and will also help you to produce the hormones which aid the uterus to finally contract down. As the uterus shrinks down the placenta is peeled off the inner lining. Blood vessels are sealed by the strong muscle fibres. The placenta flops down into the vagina and the umbilical cord ceases to pulsate and may be clamped and cut now. With a gentle contraction, the placenta eases out and is examined by the midwife. The birth is complete. You and your baby have journeyed through the gates of birth and into the courts of new life.

Jubilate Deo

1. O be joyful in the Lord, all ye lands: serve the Lord with gladness, and come before his presence with a song.
2. Be ye sure that the Lord he is God: it is he that hath made us, and not we ourselves; we are his people and the sheep of his pasture.
3. O go your way into his gates with thanksgiving, and into his courts with praise: be thankful unto him, and speak good of his name.

4. For the Lord is gracious, his mercy is everlasting: and his truth endureth from generation to generation.

Psalm 100
Book of Common Prayer

God's gift to you

So your baby's struggling journey is over. He knew the tender touch of the cradling womb for nine months, and never wanting he grew to trust, to feel secure and to love. Suddenly the trusted womb expelled him with force and passion. Now, journey ended, he needs your reassurance, your warmth, your tender touch. Hands that speak of peace and protection, hands that soothe. He needs to feel your warmth, your breathing and your skin to add to his comfort. If you lay him on his tummy on your abdomen, he will feel these things. Cover him with a towel or blanket if needed for warmth, but keep him skin to skin for these early moments if possible, for this is the womb of the spirit.

Once baby is reassured, he may open his eyes, he may stretch out his hand, and the feel of your skin speaks of rightness to him. He may look around, raise his head, turn his head from side to side. Placed near to your breast, he will root for the nipple, and when found, he will naturally take it into his mouth and suckle. There he finds comfort and satisfaction. He is at one with you again. He may now look into your eyes, and find there the light of God's countenance, the light of life. Your eyes tell him he is loved, cherished, and this is his first experience of the love of God which passes all understanding.

When your baby is born, his skin may be bluish, streaked with white grease and possibly some blood. His face is wrinkled, and his head may be moulded into a strange dome shape after its journey through the birth canal. The skin soon pinkens as he breathes, and unfolds as it meets life and love, warmth and tenderness. There needs to be quiet and calm. So often birth is met with noise, bustle, bright lights, and strong hands that intrude, all designed to terrify the baby—no wonder he screams. 'It's a boy,' someone cries out, instead of allowing mother to gently discover this for herself, and so aid acceptance of the sex of her baby. Baby has been born from mother's 'private parts' but we can be encouraged to dismiss this wonderful fact, while paradoxically we are encouraged to concentrate on the genitalia of the new baby, instead of relating first to his face, the new person. So can begin guilt for his gender, rather than graciousness for his being. Gentle discovery of the gender should be almost incidental compared to the delight of welcoming a new person into the world with a smile of wonder and face shining with love.

> The Lord bless thee and keep thee:
> The Lord make his face shine upon thee, and be gracious unto thee:
> The Lord lift up his countenance upon thee,
> And give thee peace.
> The Lord shall preserve thy going out and thy coming in
> From this time forth, and even for evermore.
> (Numbers 6:24-26; Psalm 121:8)

The birth of your baby is a climax of sensation: physically and emotionally you have been taken into extremes of effort, extremes of feelings. Now, as you cherish your baby together, you may want to laugh, cry, hug and kiss. There are no words for these precious moments. Just be yourselves, together, all three of you. Talk gently to your baby, feel him and explore his tiny naked body. Some fathers like to cut the umbilical cord at this stage, or even gently bath the baby close to the bed if the midwife is happy to allow this. Warm water may help to soothe your baby, providing there is no loss of warmth. Once back in your arms, he may be wrapped in a blanket, but if you leave his arms free they will be able to explore and caress you, feel the softness of your breast or touch your face. No intrusion or sense of hurry should be allowed to affect this cocoon of love. The midwife should quietly clear up, ensure Baby is fit and make you comfortable, then leave you together. This is your special time. You are discovering love with your child, discovering love as you become a family. Discovering love with God. It may be that you are too exhausted to feel anything very much. You may need to rest deeply before meeting your baby a little later. During this time you can feel encompassed by God's love and care for you. Allow yourself to float on this graciousness, knowing that he understands your sensitive needs, he knows your exhaustion and he blesses you with his heavenly blessing.

Perhaps Dad can enjoy holding the baby. He can begin to discover a pride, a joy and a confidence in being Father to this little one. If the midwives want to examine Baby, it is good to watch, to help, and to ask questions. Usually he is measured and weighed, his hips felt and moved, and his gripping reflex tested. His head is examined and his mouth checked to see that it is perfectly formed. There is no need to rush away at this point and make lots of telephone calls. They can wait. You need time and space for yourself, for your wife, and for your baby.

Your gift to him

So your new family falls in love together, maybe instantly, maybe gently over a few hours, or a few days. Love involves suffering, and Mum may feel a pain of separation from the baby who has evolved deep inside. You have moved, breathed and had your being totally involved with your baby for nine months. Now there is separation and loss, a dying of the 'two in one' for the resurrection of an independent being. Your body may feel empty and vacant. Suddenly the child you both dreamed of as you cherished it in pregnancy has become a reality. Perhaps he isn't as you expected, perhaps he's a different sex than you anticipated. Falling in love means getting to know each other, adjusting yourselves, your expectations, hopes and fears to the reality of the new relationship. Not only have you both become parents, but you have moved on from girlhood and boyhood, you have left behind childish things, and you now need to help each other to accept the responsibility of motherhood and fatherhood. It is a delight for the new mother to see the birth of a new father, and to feel pride and love for him. It is a delight for the new father to watch his wife as she blossoms into motherhood. It is a delight to face parenthood together, being weak and strong for each other, so that the new little baby will have security and confidence in its parents' love for him, and will grow strong as a loved, lovable and lovely person.

If there are already brothers and sisters, they need to be gently drawn into the new relationship with the baby. Knowing first and foremost that they are loved means they will have love to give to the baby. Knowing and feeling their parents' care and protection for themselves they will show care and protection for the new baby.

Just as at harvest time we offer to God all that he has given us—the ripe fruit, the perfect corn, the beautiful flowers, our work and our skills; so now you may want to offer your pregnancy and birth experience to God, and wrapped in heavenly warmth, offer your child to him. This isn't an obligatory giving away of your most precious gift to a demanding Father. The goodness and wholeness of your baby has come from an all-loving God. That God is to be found deep at the very centre of our being. The God within, the ground of our being is the God within our love for ourselves, for others, for our baby and for him. He *is* love. When we care for and love our baby we love him. When we share our homes and our lives with our baby, we share also with him. It is a continuous privilege and joy to share our lives with him, in ever-increasing wonder and praise for his abundant goodness to us and to all who trust him.

You have been privileged to have your very own Bethlehem experience. Savour its delights, its pain, its joys, its sorrows, for this is the kingdom of heaven in us and for us. Look in wonder with eyes wet with tears to him who weeps with us, bears our suffering and rejoices in our delights. Rest in his arms and feel the light of his countenance upon you, and discover his peace.

Praise and thanksgiving be to you
Lord God, heavenly Father.
We give you thanks that we have
Come through this time safely.
Thank you for midwives and doctors
And all who work and walk in your ways.
Our hearts overflow with joy and gladness
As we look with adoration on our little babe.
Knowing that all things
Begin, continue and end in you,
We commit this child into your hands,
For of such is the kingdom of heaven.
Amen.

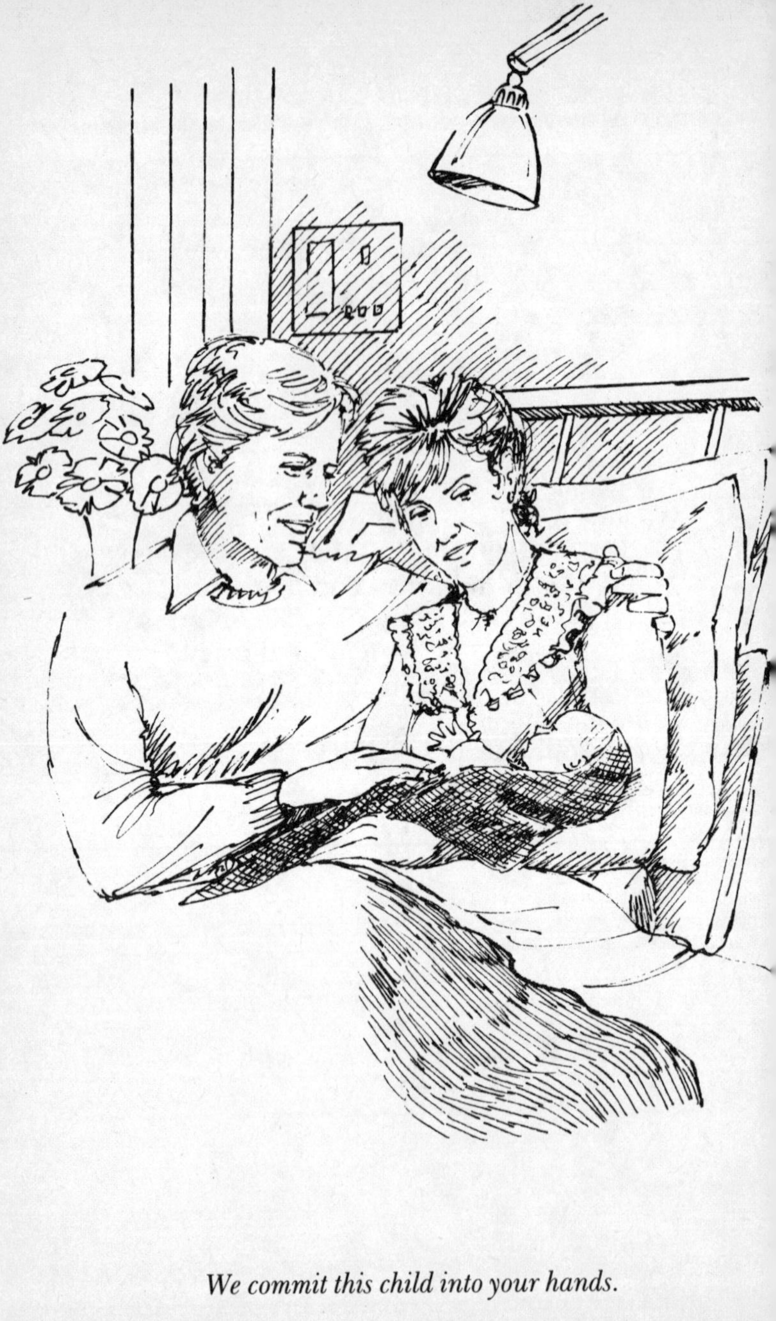

We commit this child into your hands.

CHAPTER SIX

Love in Its Tenderness

Helping you through labour
Helping your baby through labour
Caesarean birth
Special care
Prayer

YOUR LABOUR IS a uniquely personal experience. No one can predict beforehand exactly what its pattern will be. You bring into your labour not only the physical workings of your body, but also your whole personality, your past experiences of life, your joys and fears, and your relationship with your partner. It is helpful to think about what you hope for in labour, and how you think you will cope if you need help with pain or if Baby needs help to be delivered. If you and your partner have shared your thoughts and feelings through pregnancy, you will be more able to face the excitement and uncertainty of the journey through labour. You will also be ready to make informed decisions with midwives and doctors; ready to be flexible in attitude and to bring the most benefit to you and your baby. Remember that God wants you all to have a fulfilling and joyful birth day. You have learned how to help yourself by relaxation combined with special breathing and changing your position, but you may need to accept further help from the hospital. Don't be like the drowning man who refused God's help in the form of the boat and the helicopter and then got cross with him for not helping! Help is at hand, and together with the midwife and doctor you can decide which help will be best for you and your baby, and give thanks for the skill of medical staff and modern technology.

I like to show my antenatal class a picture of two plants, both with beautiful flowers. One plant is strong and straight, needing no help at all. The other plant has a lovely flower also, but it needs a stake to support it, extra fertilizer around it, added water, and a wind shield to protect it! That plant hadn't failed; it was a windy day, and it needed all the expert help the gardener could give it—then it flourished.

Helping you through labour

1. Induction

Sometimes your labour needs to be started artificially. You may have become ill, possibly with high blood pressure or some other medical problem. Alternatively the placenta may not be functioning at its best, and Baby would thrive better outside the uterus.

There are different ways of inducing labour. One of the easiest methods is the introduction of a pessary into the vagina. This slowly dissolves and releases a hormone called prostaglandis which naturally starts labour. If your cervix is ripe for labour, a pessary left to dissolve overnight may be all that is needed to start things off.

Some doctors or midwives like to break the bag of waters which surrounds the baby. This is called artificial rupture of the membrane or ARM and is performed by inserting a fine instrument, very like a crochet hook, into the vagina and through the canal in the cervix. It is usually quite painless. The release of the warm fluid changes the pressure within the uterus, and this may activate the uterus and cause contractions to begin. Once the bag of waters is broken, however, there is some risk of infection in the uterus. For this reason ARM is often combined with the use of an oxytocin drip infusion after twelve hours. Oxytocin is the hormone which causes the uterus to contract, and in this way labour can be started artificially, but there are some drawbacks to having an oxytocin drip, of which it will be helpful to be aware. You may find that because your hand is connected to a length of tubing for the drip, you are less mobile, although many mothers do walk around (so greatly helping their labour) simply by pushing the drip stand along with them! Also, you may find that contractions come far more strongly and closer together than they would naturally. You and your partner will need to be prepared to respond with your relaxation breathing and be ready for a shorter, sharper labour. While you are on an oxytocin drip, the staff may want to monitor the baby's heartbeat and your contractions, and being attached to a monitor would again make you less mobile and restricted to sitting up in bed.

You can see that once you need to divert from the natural course of labour, other problems can arise. Immobility may cause discomfort and less stimulation of the baby's head on the cervix. A shorter, sharper labour may cause you to need drugs to help with pain, or may make you too tired to cope so well. To prevent you becoming exhausted, a dextrose drip may be added to the oxytocin.

If you need to be induced either for your sake or for your baby's health, then be thankful that all this help can be given to you. However, if an induction is suggested without adequate medical reason, or simply for the convenience of the staff, then do firmly and politely question the decision, and ask that you be allowed more time to go into labour naturally.

2. Gas and oxygen (entonox)

Entonox is a mixture of nitrous oxide and oxygen. This can be breathed in through a mask or through a small mouthpiece and may be used if you are having difficulty with contractions or finding them too severe. The gas needs to be deeply inhaled as soon as the contraction starts. Once the contraction is at its peak, you can leave the gas as there is sufficient in your system to carry you through the remainder of the contraction. It is important that only you as mother hold the mask, as once you have had enough entonox your hand will naturally fall away from your face so preventing an overdose. The gas is rapidly expired through the lungs, and has no ill effects on your baby given over a limited time. You may find your lips and mouth become very dry, and sponging them with water is helpful. Some mothers find that entonox helps tremendously by taking the edge off difficult contractions, others find it makes them feel nauseated or less in control.

3. Pethidine

Pethidine is a narcotic, mood-enhancing drug with some pain relieving properties. It is administered by intramuscular injection, and takes about fifteen minutes to have effect. Many mothers feel greatly helped by pethidine because it relieves some pain, helps them to feel rather distant from the experience and may aid relaxation between contractions. Some dislike the effect of pethidine because it makes them feel confused, nauseated and detached, and breaks the concentration of their breathing pattern through contractions. If you feel the need for some help with

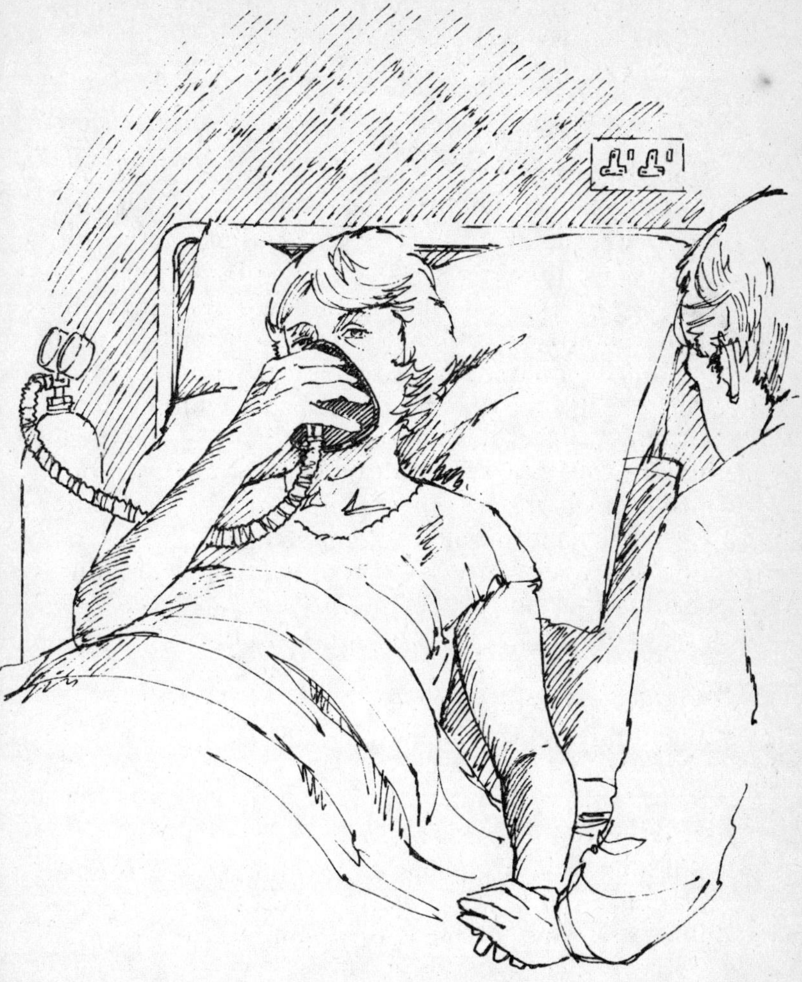

Some mothers find that Entonox helps tremendously by taking the edge off difficult contractions.

pain, it might be wise to ask for a half or even a third of the usual dose, as people do react very differently to drugs, and you may find a small dose quite sufficient.

It is vitally important to remember that the pethidine you are given passes through the placenta and into the baby's bloodstream. A small dose of pethidine for you may be a large dose for your baby. Because of this, you should not be offered pethidine during the three hours before you are expected to deliver your baby, though there is obviously a problem in that no one can be sure exactly when the birth will take place. A baby born with pethidine in his system may be slow to breathe, drowsy, floppy in muscle tone, slow to suck or so sleepy that he may miss out on that special time of awareness which a newborn babe usually has immediately after birth, and which enhances the first bonding of mother, father and baby.

4. Epidural anaesthesia

Epidural anaesthesia is an injection of local anaesthetic into the space surrounding the spinal cord in your back. It is only administered by a qualified anaesthetist and causes numbness from waist level down, thereby completely removing pain of contractions. The epidural takes about half an hour to set up and take effect. As well as relieving pain, it may cause blood pressure to fall—this being advantageous to mothers with high blood pressure. If a Caesarean section is necessary, the operation may be performed under epidural anaesthesia. The dose of anaesthetic can be topped up easily through a fine catheter left in the epidural space and strapped up onto your shoulder.

For mothers experiencing a long, difficult and

painful labour, an epidural can provide almost total relief while they remain fully conscious. However, as with most medical intervention, there are some disadvantages. Owing to the lack of sensation you will need to have a catheter passed into your bladder in order to draw off urine, and you will be restricted to bed as you cannot walk. Loss of sensation in the uterus and birth canal means you may be unaware of the urge to push in the second stage. Because of this there is a higher incidence of forceps deliveries, which also require an episiotomy. Occasionally the anaesthetic only takes effect down one side of your body causing a strange lop-sided effect. The local anaesthetic passes through the placenta and into the baby's bloodstream within ten minutes of being given. The effects on the baby are not fully understood, but there have been reports of restlessness or drowsiness after birth, depending on which anaesthetic is used for the epidural.

Making decisions about pain relief in labour may be difficult for you and the midwives. The condition of the baby is of paramount importance, and there may be other medical factors to be considered as well. Talking about the different types of pain relief and understanding their effects on you and your baby will be a great advantage. It is at this time of decision making that the quality of your relationship with the midwife or doctor is so important. You need to take the responsibility of the decision as prayerfully and carefully as possible. Any medical intervention carried out on you or your baby without your consent is an assault. By not objecting to a decision, it is assumed that consent is given. If you remain rigid in a desire for a 'natural birth', you or your baby may suffer unnecessarily, and this could have a long-term effect, such as difficulty in bonding with the child, or post-natal depression.

Hopefully you will cope well with your labour and, whether you have medical help or not, you will feel joyfully fulfilled as you adore your newborn babe together.

Helping your baby through labour

Sometimes the baby needs help to be born. Labour may have been long and Baby may become too tired or distressed. This would be apparent by the baby's heartbeat slowing down, or not picking up again between contractions. Often when a baby becomes distressed he passes some black meconium from his bowels into the surrounding fluid which should alert the midwife to assess his condition more fully. It is possible to take a tiny sample of Baby's blood before he is born—again to assess his condition. If he becomes lodged in an awkward position it may be necessary to perform a Caesarean section in which he is born through a cut in the mother's abdomen. Sometimes it is possible to help the baby out of the birth canal by the use of forceps, lifting him gently out. Other times, all that is needed is a cut, or episiotomy, made in the birth outlet, so allowing more room for the baby's head to be born without further delay.

1. Episiotomy

An episiotomy is a cut made with scissors by the midwife through the thin stretched tissues of the birth outlet. It is done to prevent long delays and the mother's tissues from being torn during birth—if it is thought that the tear might be severe. A few years ago almost every mother had an episiotomy but now it is hopefully only done if thought really essential. You should be told that an episiotomy will be performed and your agreement obtained. The midwife may inject the tissues of the perineum, just below the birth outlet, with a local anaesthetic or she may make the episiotomy at the height of a contraction, when the tissues are so stretched around the baby's head that there is little or no sensation, and mothers are often quite unaware that a cut has been made. Once the episiotomy is made the baby is usually born with ease.

The episiotomy has to be stitched up very carefully soon after the birth. Some mothers feel this is such an anticlimax after the birth of the baby, and are very anxious that being stitched will hurt. It is so necessary that your partner stays with you now, if you wish, with the new baby still close by. Your legs will need to go up into stirrups, but don't allow this to be done until just before the doctor is ready as you may get shaky or cold. Once ready, the doctor will inject you with local anaesthetic around the episiotomy. Do make absolutely sure that the anaesthetic has taken full effect before the doctor begins to stitch. You should feel no pain, and if you do, say so, and continue to complain until more anaesthetic is put in. Your partner can help by speaking up for you at this time. It is essential that you feel no pain, so that you are relaxed and the delicate layers of muscle and skin can be stitched carefully and well. This is important for your future health—for complete healing of the pelvic floor, to restore full muscle tone, and to help you to know that your enjoyment of a normal sexual relationship is not affected.

The stitches will naturally dissolve over the following days, and you will need to take care in keeping the area clean and free from infection. You may feel sore, so help yourself by sitting on a rubber ring, or special cushion. When you first have your bowels open after an episiotomy it is helpful to press a sanitary towel over the stitches to relieve discomfort. Some hospitals recommend daily salt baths, or heat treatment by lamps, to promote healing.

2. Forceps delivery

The thought of a forceps delivery causes some couples a lot of anxiety, but it really need not do so. Forceps are like stainless steel salad servers especially designed so that they cannot cause undue pressure on the baby's head. Forceps may be needed if the uterus becomes too tired to finally push the baby out once just inside the vagina, or if the baby has become too tired and it is thought best to help him out into the world. The situation should be discussed with you, and if you are unsure about the reasons why forceps are being suggested, then do ask and make sure you understand and agree. It is a doctor's decision, and only a doctor will perform a forceps delivery. Having agreed this is the best course of action for you and your baby, an episiotomy will be performed. Next, the doctor will slip one blade of the forceps at a time into the vagina around the baby's head. The two blades then lock apart so that they are unable to put too great a pressure on the baby's head which is now gently cradled in the forceps. With the next contraction, the doctor gently eases the head out of the vagina and your baby is born. It is often a great relief to parents and Baby that the birth is over and the joy of welcoming the babe will overcome any sense of disappointment that forceps were needed.

Caesarean birth

A Caesarean section is an operation, performed under

a general or epidural anaesthetic, in which the baby is delivered through a cut made in the abdominal wall into the uterus.

There are various reasons why a Caesarean section may be needed. One of the most common is that the baby's head is not able to pass through the mother's pelvis. This is called disproportion and may occur in very small, short mothers. These days doctors often prefer to deliver breech babies by Caesarean section as they feel there is less risk to the baby. If an ultrasound scan shows the placenta is lying very low in the uterus, or even across the cervix (*placenta previa*), then a Caesarean section is imperative as there could be severe haemorrhaging with a vaginal delivery.

A Caesarean section may be undertaken as an emergency during labour if the baby becomes seriously distressed, or the doctors are concerned for the mother's health. The fact that you have had a Caesarean section once does not mean that you cannot deliver another baby vaginally. Most doctors will be happy to give you a trial of labour and be ready to go ahead with the Caesarean section only if it is needed.

If you need a Caesarean section you will be given a pubic shave, and a catheter will be inserted into your bladder to draw off any urine. You will be given a short-lasting general anaesthetic, or an epidural anaesthetic if you agree. The latter has the advantage that you will be able to enjoy the birth of your baby and watch the delivery if you wish, and you will not suffer from the usual after effects of an operation, such as drowsiness or nausea.

There is an excited air of expectancy then relief in the theatre when a Caesarean section is performed. The operation may last only a few minutes before the baby is delivered gently through the 'bikini line' incision in the abdominal wall. It is thrilling for everyone there to see a baby, which may have caused real anxiety during labour, being delivered safe and well. A paediatrician checks the baby and, providing all *is* well, may allow the father to hold and cuddle the newborn infant. Some doctors will allow fathers to stay in the theatre during the operation. It is certainly worth asking, if that is what you both want. The abdominal incision is closed in separate layers with self-dissolving stitches and the final skin stitches will be left in for a week before being taken out.

Following a Caesarean section you would expect to remain in hospital for at least a week, receiving special nursing care. It is important to move around to aid normal circulation. There is no reason why you should not breastfeed your baby if you so wish, and placing the baby on a pillow alongside you to feed will avoid any extra pressure being put on your abdomen as the wound heals.

You may feel a little disappointed, or even feel that things went wrong, after having a Caesarean section. This is a natural enough reaction, and hopefully you may be able to have a normal vaginal delivery if there is to be a next time. Try to think how incredibly fortunate you and your baby are that there was what may have been a life-saving operation available. Thank God for doctors, nurses and modern technology, for education and civilization, for your baby, alive and hopefully well and ready to thrive. Thank God for the love which surrounds you, your partner and your babe. Things didn't go wrong—they went right, following some serious problem. Let us rejoice and be glad!

Special care

If your baby is premature or very small he may need

special intensive nursing and medical care to help him through the early days. A tiny baby may need help to breathe, so oxygen may be given for a while, or continuously until he has become stronger. A tiny or weak baby will need careful feeding. It is best if the baby can suckle from his mother, but if he is too weak he may be fed breast milk through a fine catheter which is passed through his nose and into his stomach. A baby requiring special care needs to be kept warm at a controlled temperature and may be placed in an incubator. If your baby needs special care, you may feel very anxious and somehow inadequate that you cannot care for him yourself. Ask as many questions as you can and find out what the problem is and what is being done about it. It may be that Baby was simply very tired after delivery, or that he has some slight medical problem or small abnormality, or maybe he is more seriously ill and failing to thrive. If you don't know exactly what is wrong you may fear something far worse. Insist on knowing, understanding and, above all, on being with your baby if at all possible. Most special care units value the parents being with the sick baby for they know that alongside the medical care, Baby needs your care, your touch, your loving eyes, to help give him the love and warmth for life that he needs. Surround your baby with prayer, with hope, with love. You cannot do better. Entrust him into the skilled hands of doctors and nurses. Pray that whatever the outcome nothing but good will come from the experience. It may seem inconceivable that good can come from such anxiety, but this is the stuff that miracles are made of, this is the redemption that only God brings from a time of trial.

Heavenly Father, we have walked
Along a troubled pathway,
Yet we have experienced
Your love, encouragement and skill,
And now rejoice that all will be well.
Thank you for showing us that if
We put our trust in you
We may discover unnumbered blessings
Like stars against a darkened sky.
We ask that through our problems
Love will be deeper, richer and closer.
Lord, in your mercy, hear our prayer.
Amen.

CHAPTER SEVEN

Hope for Our Fear

For those of you enjoying a happy, healthy pregnancy, it may be tempting to miss out this chapter and to avoid the pain it may bring. Fears of miscarriage, or of having a stillborn baby, may be fears that are quickly passed over and forgotten. Yet these very fears may nag at you sometimes during the night, or possibly come in a dream which disturbs you. Most expectant parents have wondered how they would cope if their precious little one died either before, during or after birth. I would like you to read on, because if you face a fear fully, you can help yourself to cope with it more positively, rather than letting it linger on half unnoticed. It could be that a friend, neighbour or relative will experience the sad loss of a baby and, having understood a little about it, you could be in a stronger position to come alongside the grieving couple and be a support and comfort in their crisis.

Before reading further about miscarriage or the birth of a stillborn babe, look at these words written by a hymn-writer earlier this century:

> God is love: and he enfoldeth
>   all the world in one embrace;
> With unfailing grasp he holdeth

every child of every race.
And when human hearts are breaking
under sorrow's iron rod,
Then they find that self-same aching
deep within the heart of God.

Timothy Rees

Those last two lines are full of such truth. God grieves with us in our tragedies. God weeps with us in our loss. He does not pick out certain babies to die, or certain parents to punish—what an impossibly dreadful Father that would be! He wants life, love, health and joy for each and every one, and wants it more abundantly, until our cup flows over with goodness and richness of love for him, for one another and for ourselves. This is the kingdom of heaven. Yet he allowed the risk of humanity, rather than an artificial perfection. He allowed the risk of our free will. He allowed for the possibility of failure, of disease. He allowed for us the freedom to accept or to reject him. This is his majesty, his love for us, so great that there is freedom, not dictatorship; captivation, not captivity. He rejoices in our joys and delights. He aches for our pains and sorrows. If you grieve for a little one, you grieve because you love and have lost. How much more our heavenly Father loves and grieves. Yet it is love that wins through. It is love which heals. It is love which is inextinguishable, and it is that love in our hearts that is the Christ within.

When pregnancy fails

I have deliberately used this heading as it is the title of a book written by Susan Borg and Judith Lasker, published by Routledge and Kegan Paul. It is a book highly recommended for any couple facing the sad

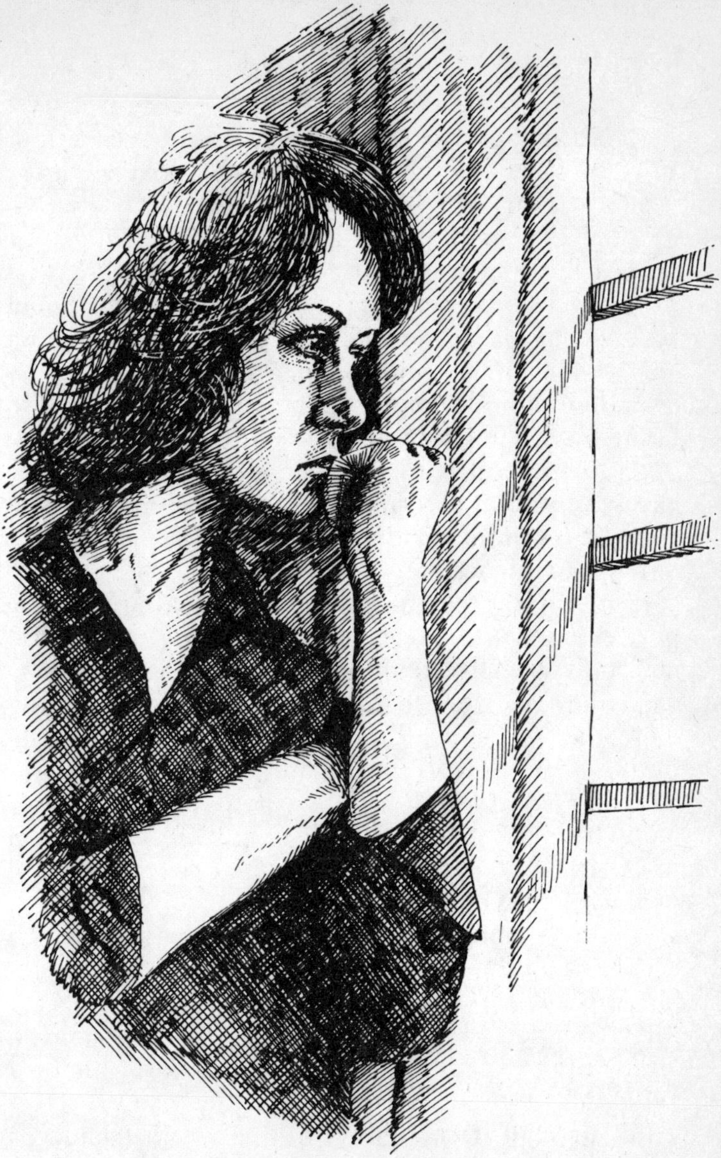

It is love which heals.

bewilderment of miscarriage, stillbirth or infant death.

A miscarriage occurs in fifteen to twenty per cent of all conceptions. When this happens before the baby is capable of surviving (around the twenty-fourth week) it is called a 'spontaneous abortion'. Seventy-five per cent of these spontaneous abortions occur in the first twelve weeks of pregnancy, often before the woman realizes she is pregnant. These are due either to an abnormality in the embryo or in the process of its implantation in the uterus. These abortions may also occur because of serious disease in the mother, malnutrition, exposure to toxic chemicals, drugs, X-rays, excessive smoking or high alcohol consumption. The risk of a spontaneous abortion is greater if a mother is in her late thirties.

If in early pregnancy you become aware of low period-like pains, a heavy full feeling, or actual pain, you may be threatening to miscarry. There may either be some very slight or more apparent bleeding from the vagina. If this occurs, go to bed and telephone your doctor immediately. Sometimes slight bleeding occurs each month when you would normally have had a period. This simply means the level of hormones is not quite right and can be rectified with injections of extra progesterone.

An 'inevitable abortion' is a miscarriage which occurs when the baby has already died. Sadly there is nothing you can do in this situation and your doctor will advise you whether it is best for you to deliver the little embryo vaginally, or whether removal under a general anaesthetic is needed.

Miscarriage after the twelfth week of pregnancy is far less common. Sometimes the cervix is weak or incompetent and begins to dilate far too early. This can sometimes be put right by the insertion of a stitch through the cervix which literally holds it shut.

A miscarriage after the twentieth week of pregnancy may mean that the placenta has ceased to function properly. If a miscarriage of this nature is threatened, bed rest and an excellent diet may help to save the baby.

The fact that you have had one or more miscarriages does not necessarily mean you cannot have a normal, healthy pregnancy and a live baby another time, although your chances of miscarriage remain higher than normal. In view of this, do discuss the situation with your doctor before you become pregnant again, so that he and you can plan ahead how best to maintain the pregnancy and to help you to have the baby you so long for.

The grief experienced by couples who have had a miscarriage is one of the least understood griefs. It is as if society just can't take miscarriage seriously. Doctors, nurses, neighbours, people in the street seem to quickly dismiss the emotional, spiritual and physical trauma with a quick remark like: 'Oh, forget it, you can have another baby,' or: 'It's nature's way of getting rid of imperfect babies,' or: 'Never mind, you're young and healthy.' Yet for the couple there is first the shock of the actual abortion. Many women experience heavy bleeding with painful contractions and the expulsion of a tiny but often recognizable foetus—an experience not easily forgotten. There is the sense of failure among friends and colleagues, an awkwardness in conversation. Constantly couples may wonder if they should have gone to that party, had a drink, or made love. None of these things need be relevant, but they become questions of great importance. There may be a sense of guilt. Perhaps they had felt a little ambivalent towards the pregnancy in the first place.

For most couples the embryo, even in the first month or two of pregnancy, had already become a real baby—a little person with a name and personality. There is all the fantasy and expectations of parents to be. When there is a late miscarriage, the couple had perhaps grown accustomed to feeling their baby kicking and moving, sleeping or wriggling. Now there is emptiness, loss. There is the need to remember all the little details of planned care—the baby clothes, the nursery, the toys—and to allow time and space to grieve for the lost little one; to comfort and love each other through this poorly-understood sorrow, and then gently to learn to face the future again with hope.

When a baby dies

When a baby dies shortly before it is born, the mother may sense something is wrong. The baby's movements would have ceased, and there would be no foetal heart sounds heard by midwife or doctor. Blood tests or a scan may provide further evidence, and the couple will gradually realize that their worst fears are confirmed. The hopelessness and sense of failure can be shattering. Now the little still baby has to be delivered. This is often by means of an induced labour, or occasionally by Caesarean section. All the effort of labour now seems wasted, the feeling of creativity gone. There is a double loss, the loss of the live baby so hoped for, and the physical loss of the baby from the mother's body. There is time to adapt a little to the tragedy, time to realize that hope is lost for this baby's life, time to go over the questions: why did it happen? How did it happen? What now?

For some couples there is the loss of a baby at birth. Birth and death come together, hand in hand. For some reason the baby fails to survive the journey of birth. The natural excitement of labour suddenly becomes full of anxiety as midwives and doctors realize that the baby is distressed. A Caesarean section may be performed, or the mother may deliver the little one who is still and does not breathe despite attempts to stimulate him. It is a profound shock. Tired, shocked and numbed the realization of what has happened gradually dawns, and the couple begin a time of questioning, of grieving.

When a baby dies just before, or during birth, it may help if you can hold him. Until recent times it was felt to be less distressing for the mother if the baby was quickly and quietly removed. Yet mothers and fathers have said how they wish so much that they had seen their baby, known what he looked like, and seen that he was beautiful, looking as if simply sleeping. Without seeing the baby, the imagination can conjure up dreadful pictures of deformed monsters which can add enormous distress to the grieving couple. Parents love their baby, even if stillborn, and in their acute distress they can find comfort in holding, kissing, caressing and cuddling him before finally saying farewell. If you, or the hospital staff, can take a picture of your baby, this may help over the coming months. You both knew your baby as a real little person, you lived together for nine months. You have memories, and a picture will help you to know that he wasn't some kind of fantasy to be brushed aside. Your baby was real.

Try to keep a little memento of your baby, a shawl or fluffy toy you had ready. Again, although this seems almost too sad to contemplate, it will help you to be able to touch them, to know he was real. You grieve the loss of a real baby. Your grief is legitimate, and you will need time and comfort before the hurt becomes easier to bear. The hospital staff should help you to make any arrangements for a funeral. A little grave or a marked place in a cemetery or garden will enable you to have a focus for your grief.

Over the following days you can gradually ask more about how and why your baby died. It is important to know the reasons, to help you piece together this shattering experience. You may feel angry that more could not have been done to help your baby; angry at yourselves for not producing a live baby; angry even at your baby for not surviving. These are all completely natural feelings, and it can only be good to express them, over and over again, if need be, to a close friend or to each other as you gently come to accept the reality of death.

After a day or two, the mother's milk will fill her breasts and this fullness will only serve to make her loss more painful, but treatment can be given to suppress the flow of milk. Relatives and friends now need to come alongside, gently and carefully. Remarks such as: 'You can have another baby,' or, 'It's nature's way of being kind,' and, 'You'll get over it,' serve only to dismiss the reality of grief, and the ardent seeking of a positive outcome is seldom appreciated. Leaving the hospital with empty arms may be agony, and coming home to an empty nursery will need all the love, care and crying together necessary to gradually ease your burden. You may never forget the little one you lost. The pain may never completely leave you, but time, love and acceptance will gently heal the hurt and enable you to look forward bravely together again.

It may be that your baby is born alive, but very frail and weak, and is unable to survive more than a few hours, days or weeks. For parents of such a child these are times of anguish. The tiring yet joyful labour is over, but your joy is tainted with the realization that your babe is very sick. He may be quickly removed to the special care baby unit, or even rapidly transferred to a different hospital where facilities are better fitted for his needs. In both instances you may have had little time to hold and get to know your baby. Many special care baby units now have sleeping accommodation for Mother, which is ideal—if only they could have family units where Father could stay as well. It is important to ask that you can be taken to be with your baby, and if possible to breastfeed or supply breast milk for feeding. It is understood at special care units how vital it is for both mother and child to be in close physical contact, even if the baby is in an incubator. This time of acute anxiety, of hopes and fears, may feel like some kind of hell. Minute by minute you hope, you pray. The last words of nurse or doctor become a lifeline to you. The uncertainty of the situation can be almost unbearable. Do you send out birth announcement cards? What do you tell friends and relatives? You may wonder what you have done wrong for your child to be failing, and you may feel you are being punished. Father carries a heavy load of responsibility being concerned for Mother's health and wellbeing, and desperately hoping Baby will survive. At this time of real anguish, parents can meet together in the special care unit and be of mutual support and comfort. The staff should help you to cope with and express your anxieties, your hopes and fears. As you help to nurse your sick baby, so you can feel you are a real mother and father to this frail tiny person. You may feel almost afraid to love the baby too much, knowing you may have to part. These few days or weeks are very, very special. They are the lifetime of your baby, however short. They are the days of the tangible reality of love for your babe, and for you as parents. A time of love, hope, care and comfort.

Comfort thy sorrows

Falling in love, getting married, going on honeymoon, living together as a young couple so much in love, the excitement of expecting your first child, are all part of the romance of life in which family and friends share your happiness and hopes for the future. The death of a baby is a painful affront to those shared hopes, a tragedy which gate crashes into life. Unwanted, unacceptable, unsociable. Happiness becomes heaviness, delight turns to despair, and grief may pervade every aspect of life. Yet grief itself is where healing of the hurt begins. A young couple may have had little time to consolidate their marriage relationship, and in their grief will need to reassure and be reassured of their love for each other. Grief is lonely and unique, and it is so necessary that you talk openly about your feelings. There should be no wall, no barrier, against expressing grief differently and trying to cope in very different ways. A husband may feel it is better not to say too much, to remind each other of the loss; a wife may be longing to talk about each and every detail of their baby, of memories, hopes and fantasies for the future.

Your relationship, your love for each other, will almost inevitably change now, and can be greatly strengthened and deepened. Try to talk each day about your feelings, cry together, hold and hug each other. You may feel the need for someone to share this time with you—a close friend, or relative, or a minister or doctor you trust. You may feel angry, guilty or that people were to blame for the death. You will need to express your thoughts and feelings over and over again, and make some sense, order and reason out of the nonsense, disorder and unreasonability of your infant's untimely death. Both of you may be physically very tired, and Mother will need to heal after the labour or Caesarean section. You really will need to 'comfort thy sorrows' for and with each other and you may eventually discover a new value for life, a new value for each other, your marriage, your present or future children, and your love.

Friends and family may feel a confusion in their sorrow. Was it birth or death? Is this now bereavement, or a time to be rapidly forgotten? Are the couple parents or not? This sense of confusion can bring about a conspiracy of silence, an embarrassment, which will not help the grieving parents. Friends and relatives do care and need to show their caring by being alongside the couple, either to listen, to hold, to help in practical ways, or simply to be there for them. It is good and necessary to grieve. Grief left to smoulder silently deep inside can lead to a solid depression which may continue right through life. Grieving parents won't ever forget. They will remember the birthday each year, think of their lost child over the years—starting school, growing up into life—yet the emptiness will lose its anguish, and will lose its pain. Other children may be born and their happiness will spill over into the dark area of memories and will help to create the true harmony in life's melody with its major and minor keys. Love overcomes death, and new hope rises gently over the horizon of loss like the first faltering rays of the morning sun kiss the tearful dewdrops with warmth.

Answer thy prayerfulness

The death of a baby is a tragedy, and no one should

underestimate the grief and suffering that accompanies it. The depth of grief reflects the degree of love felt for the little one. That depth of love is God. Right there at the very centre of your grief is God, grieving with you. If you try to turn away from the pain you may miss a closer walk with him. If you choose to deny the hurt, you may only replace it with hardness. Somehow, through prayer, and only by God's grace, a miracle occurs, and you are enabled to say yes to the hurt, yes to the dark fears, yes to the loss.

When we can accept grief and go with it, we can discover something new in our lives. It is the realization that we are deeper, richer, fuller people because of facing our anguish. We discover new strengths we never imagined possible. We find that death has brought alive those hidden dormant parts of our spirits of which we were previously unaware. We discover the Christ within. The suffering, loving, accepting Christ with whom it is our privilege to be friends. This new discovery will not be heralded by a fanfare, we will not suddenly be told we have found new possibilities. It may come as a fine glimmer of light, of hope. It may come tentatively, sensitively, tiptoeing into our prayers, our thoughts, our memories and relationships. There, before us, perhaps for a fleeting moment will be the new hope which is Christ. Gently and gradually, in our own time, that glimmer of hope will grow and a new dawn will break into our hearts. Because we have been willing to feel our pain, to despair over the unreasonableness of it all, so we shall receive new life and new love by the gift of his grace to us. When in our prayers we can be utterly honest and admit we care and yet don't care, love and yet don't love, believe and yet do not believe, then we find God, and share in his suffering and his love as he shares in ours. It simply means being me with him.

As change occurs over the following weeks, months and years you may find you place new value on your lives, your relationships, your children. Beliefs may be firmer, more secure. You may find you share a far deeper understanding for others who suffer in some way, whether it be loss or sickness or depression. Gradually you will find a new sense of wellbeing and confidence. Healing may be slow, but scars need not be ugly, they can be signs of deeper love and care for ourselves, for each other and for God.

As Harry Williams writes,

> For God makes of a loss that is real and devastating the means of an increased apprehension of Himself, which is our only ultimate gain—though that is a truth that it may take years or a lifetime to realise. [*The Joy of God*, Mitchell Beasley, page 66.]

For some reason life was not to be for your little one. I love the verse in Matthew's Gospel which speaks of their angels, and I feel it can bring comfort and reassurance to you now: 'Take heed that ye despise not one of these little ones; for I say unto you, that in heaven their angels do always behold the face of my Father which is in heaven' (Matthew 18:10).

Father, we have loved and lost.
Our hearts ache with sadness and grief.
Accept our pain, our tears, our sorrow.
Hold us closely in your arms
So that we may learn that
Our emptiness shall be filled,
Our pain soothed, and our eyes opened
To behold your infinite compassion and care.
Help us to share our loss together
So that we may help one another
To turn our weakness into strength,
And our loss into courage.
Through Jesus Christ, our risen Lord.
Amen.

CHAPTER EIGHT

Mornings of Joy

Preparation for breastfeeding
Early days
Enjoying breastfeeding
The light of his countenance
Prayer

FOR MANY WOMEN the desire to breastfeed is almost as strong as the desire to have a baby. It is the most basic natural expression of love and care for your baby. Breast is best, and if you want to breastfeed there is almost never any reason why you shouldn't. There are only a handful of very serious medical conditions or treatments which might prohibit breastfeeding. The shape or size of your breasts is of no concern. The only reason for bottle feeding is because you want to, or you feel you've breastfed for long enough, or plan to return to work. You may be unsure during your pregnancy whether you want to breastfeed or not, and it is worth discussing this with your partner. Sometimes a difficult relationship with your own parents might colour your attitude about feeding, or feeling in some sense that breastfeeding is almost animal like. Negative remarks about breastfeeding may be voiced by someone who didn't breastfeed her own babies for various reasons, there can even be a touch of jealousy. It can be hard for a couple to free themselves from such influences, but I hope you can think of yourselves as free to make your own decision and fully confident in the ability of your exquisitely

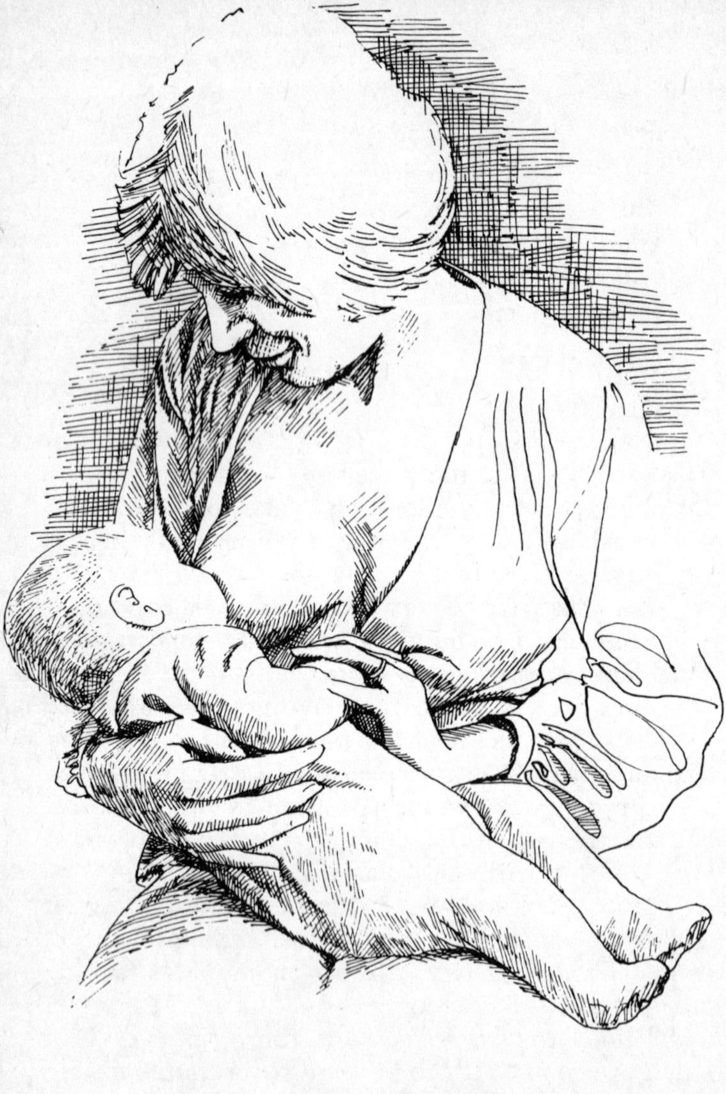

It is the most basic natural expression of love and care for your baby.

made body to produce not only your baby, but milk to feed, and love to cherish, one of God's little ones.

Preparation for breastfeeding

There is no preparation you need make for your breasts to breastfeed. Nature provides oil to soften the skin from little glands on the areola—the dark area around the nipple. It is important not to wash this oil off with soap, just bathe the breasts with warm water. The hormones of pregnancy will soften and enlarge your breasts, and there will be a yellowish fluid called colostrum in the breasts until two or three days after the baby is born. This colostrum is the bridging fluid for the baby between the placental fluid and true breast milk. It is very rich in protein, and has antibodies which prevent infection. It coats the lining of Baby's intestine with a protective layer against invading bacteria. It is non-allergenic. Frequent small feeds help to break down bilirubin in the liver and so prevent jaundice in the newborn. You can see that colostrum is the most perfect substance for a baby and because of its high protein content only a little is needed. There is no need to express any colostrum from the breasts before baby is born.

It is helpful if you can prepare yourselves for breastfeeding. Talk together about how you feel towards it. Discuss the social aspects—are you going to avoid social activities while breastfeeding, or simply take your baby along with you? How do you feel about feeding in public? I think breastfeeding can be somewhat over-romanticized with pictures of beautiful semi-naked women doting over their naked infant through a haze of sunshine! Actually breastfeeding can be a very practical affair. You can feed almost unnoticed in a crowd—a pullover is easiest to wear and then you can tuck Baby up close to you and no one will notice. I'm not suggesting you hide the fact you are feeding, but somewhere there is a compromise between what could be embarrassing for some and what is natural for others. It is good if you can both attend antenatal classes at your local hospital so that you can learn together about breastfeeding. The National Childbirth Trust have trained breastfeeding counsellors attached to antenatal classes in most areas. They will provide detailed information about feeding, and are available on a twenty-four-hour basis to help with any non-medical breastfeeding difficulties which you might encounter, and to give you reassurance and encouragement over the coming months.

When you first arrive home with your new baby, you will need rest and quiet so that all three of you can relax and devote peaceful time to feeding and cuddling your baby. Too many visitors and too much housework and cooking can all disrupt this peace which is so necessary until breastfeeding is established. Because of this it is wise to plan ahead. Have plenty of meals in the freezer, or know where the nearest take-away is, and be firm about the number of visitors you have, quietly insisting they don't stay too long. If friends want to help, the best thing they can do is to take the ironing, bake a pie, or have your toddler for a while—but leave Mother, Father and Baby quietly alone during this precious time.

Early days

If you are having your baby in hospital do make sure the nurses know that you wish to breastfeed him totally, or you may find he is given a bottle of dextrose or milk by an overkeen night nurse!

Once you have safely given birth to your little one, you may like to suckle him at your breast during the first hour. This is the best possible thing to do as the baby's sucking reflex is very strong—some babies are born sucking, eagerly seeking the breast. Baby is very awake and aware during this first hour, providing pethidine has not recently been given to the mother. It is also possible to suckle your baby very soon after a Caesarean section if you put him on a pillow under your arm to relieve pressure on your abdomen. The nurses will help and encourage you.

During the first two or three days it is good not to set a limit on the amount of sucking and little feeds your baby has. Forget all about clocks and simply feed any time either you or your baby want to. Hold him with his tummy against your tummy so he doesn't have to twist his neck and cause a drag on the nipple which could make it sore. Make sure that all of the nipple and areola are in baby's mouth. Some soreness is very common in the early days, and to limit feeding only frustrates you both and delays the soreness until a day or two later. If you feel sore, expose the breasts to the air as much as possible and don't use any waterproof backed pads for leaking as these make the skin soggy and more liable to soreness. A man's handkerchief with a one-way nappy liner is a good guard against leaking. Soreness usually passes off within a day or two, but do seek prompt advice from your breastfeeding counsellor if you have any type of problem. There are few problems which can't be overcome if you really want to breastfeed.

When your baby sucks, the stimulation of the breast causes hormones to be released which then produce milk. After a few seconds you may be aware of a full tingling sensation called the let-down reflex. This is milk actually being supplied to your baby. You need to allow time for this to happen, so never rush a feed. Tension or anxiety can inhibit the let-down reflex. As breastfeeding becomes established, so even the thought of your baby can promote the let-down reflex.

During the first two to four days after the birth, the baby will suckle colostrum which is so vital for health. The milk will then come into the breasts, and this, plus an increased blood supply, can make the breasts feel very full and hard for a day or two. This is called engorgement and is quite natural. Simply give your baby small feeds frequently. Mothers were at one time told to feed ten minutes each side every four hours! This leads to painful engorgement, crying babies wanting a feed or cuddle, and tense, distressed mothers! Don't be told by anyone when to feed your baby, simply follow your own intuition, instincts and maternal feelings—they're all there, so tune in to those feelings and use them. You are the best mother in the world for your baby and don't allow anyone to sow even a seed of doubt in your mind.

As the hormones stimulate the production of milk when you suckle, so those same hormones help to contract the muscles of the uterus. (This is an excellent reason for feeding very soon after birth, as it can aid the natural expulsion of the placenta.) You may feel this contracting of the uterus as 'after pains'. Deep breathing and relaxation will help you over these pains which will pass off within a week or two. It is good to know that breastfeeding is helping your body to return to normal.

Enjoying breastfeeding

After the first week or two, you will see that your baby has established some sort of pattern to his day. He may feed more at certain times, sleep or want to play and be cuddled at other times. You will need to rest as much as possible and have plenty of help at home. As you both love and care for your baby, so you will both need to love and care for each other. When Mum feeds Baby, it is a good time for Dad to make a warm drink and to stay alongside to encourage and adore both Mother and child.

Between feeds, try to treat yourself to a favourite snack and drink, because it's not only good to keep your physical energy up, but it gives you a necessary psychological boost. The more you nurse the nursing, mother the mothering, and care for the caring, the better. You need 600-800 extra calories while breastfeeding, but it is sufficient to eat a sensible diet according to hunger. Drink according to thirst, not allowing yourself to go thirsty. Remember that whatever you take into your body goes through the milk to your baby. That applies to alcohol as well so it would be wise to be very moderate. Only take drugs prescribed by your doctor, who knows you are breastfeeding, and never take 'over the counter' drugs—not even cough mixtures. If you are considering birth control, you should know that the pill does reduce your supply of milk, and even the mini pill may give your baby extra hormones. It would be best to seek advice from your Family Planning Clinic or a doctor who knows you are breastfeeding and that you wish to continue to do so.

For several weeks you will probably be feeding your baby once or twice during the night. Try to resolve yourself to this fact, or you may find yourself constantly fighting the night feed and it becoming a source of upset. These weeks may seem long to you at the time, but they're not really and soon pass. Make night feeds easy. Have your baby either in bed with you, or very close by in a crib. You can feed lying down and if your baby is in bed with you, he will latch on to your breast quite naturally when he wants a feed. There is no need to always change his nappy during the night, unless very soiled. One-way nappy liners should increase his comfort. You can invest in some thick nappies and plastic pants and leave the changing till morning. After all, once he is sleeping through the night he won't have a nappy change until morning!

If you are becoming overtired, depressed, or trying to cope with a problem, the night feed can find you at your lowest. I can remember feeling I was the only woman in the world breastfeeding a baby at 3 a.m.! Try to comfort yourself, or perhaps Dad will make a cup of tea for you and for himself, and give you a hug which is just as important. It isn't always easy, but most mothers find this quiet night feed a wonderful chance to adore their little one without any hurry or distraction, especially if there are other young children to cope with during the day.

If there are other children, or a young toddler, it helps if you can manage to occupy them while you feed the baby—perhaps with a jigsaw, the television or a story. The toddler needs some kind of preparation for your breastfeeding the new baby, so showing him some pictures or talking about breastfeeding can be useful. Best of all, take him to a friend of yours who is breastfeeding, so it becomes just a normal part of everyday life.

You will know when breastfeeding is going well. Baby will thrive and will look healthy and happy. There will be a good pattern of feeding and sleeping, cuddling and playing. There will be at least six wet nappies a day, and stools will be soft and golden yellow. Weight gain will vary enormously, but you will see that your baby is gaining and developing normally. Try not to become obsessed with weight unless there is a definite problem. There are natural growth spurts, often at about six and twelve weeks, when your baby may become more hungry than usual. You will simply need to increase your milk supply by feeding a little more often for a few days. Follow your instincts and if you need help, contact a responsible breastfeeding counsellor. Some doctors or health visitors may be quick to advise bottle feeding, but if this is against all you had hoped for, it can be a source of regret for years to come. Some baby clinics can cause more upset than reassurance with an obsession over weight gain and with anxious mothers comparing their babies. Many a mother has left the clinic in tears! Other clinics sensibly allow for the very different rate at which babies grow and develop, and help the young mother to feel confident in her ability to feed and nurture her child.

Lack of self-confidence and other people's remarks and attitudes can be your worst enemies! At some hospitals every breastfeeding mother is given a sample of formula baby feed as a promotional gimmick from the commercial companies 'just in case you need it'. This can instil a sense of possible failure into a mother who wants to breastfeed before she's even tried—a practice I would like to see stopped.

As a young couple you need to relax and enjoy breastfeeding. Being confident in your ability to feed your baby as and when and where you wish, you can protect each other from the doubts, loss of confidence and mass advertising which only serve to undermine that confidence.

The light of his countenance

When your baby was born the love you had for him was shown by the look of adoration on your face, by your smile and the light in your eyes—this was the light of your countenance. I make no apologies for writing this blessing again:

> The Lord bless thee and keep thee:
> The Lord make his face shine upon thee,
> and be gracious unto thee:
> The Lord lift up his countenance upon thee,
> And give thee peace.
> The Lord shall preserve thy going out and
> thy coming in
> From this time forth, and even for evermore.
> (Numbers 6:24–26; Psalm 121:8)

Each time you feed your baby and look lovingly and adoringly at him, you give him this blessing on God's behalf. You represent God to your baby, for he knows of no other experience so consistently in his little life than being held and loved by you, his earthly mother and father. I believe his experience of love and care with you will enable him to paint a picture of the face of God as he grows up—and God's face will be smiling, full of love. If you feel loved yourself, by your parents, by your partner, by God, you will be able to show that same love to your child. Your love will not possess, your arms will not clutch for your own sake, desperately needing your baby to love you because you are empty. That is the possessive love which destroys. God's love is gracious.

> Love suffereth long, and is kind; love envieth
> not; love vaunteth not itself, is not puffed up.
> Doth not behave itself unseemly, seeketh not her own,
> is not easily provoked, thinketh no evil;

Rejoiceth not in iniquity, but rejoiceth in
the truth;
Beareth all things, believeth all things, hopeth all
things, endureth all things.
Love never faileth.

(1 Corinthians 13:4-8, substituting 'love' for 'charity'.)

Can we, as mothers, reach such a standard of love as this? It seems a hard task, however much we love our children, yet it is also the easiest and most natural thing in the world. When you hold your baby and gently caress him, when you feel him at the breast, or close to you with skin-to-skin contact, when you look into his eyes with wonder and love, when you smile in sheer delight for his sake, then you are an ambassador for Christ and you show your baby what true love, God's love, is all about. Over the days, weeks and months, your baby grows to feel loved, secure and fed. For he is fed with spiritual food as well as physical food. He is fed the warmth of love, of contact, as well as the milk of human kindness. Gradually he builds up a picture of himself as someone who is sure of love, and the beginnings of a confident 'I am' become the basis of a healthy self-love, self-affirmation. This is the womb of the spirit, an experience of God which will spread out to others. It will be easy for him to believe in a loving God as he is physically handled as well as fed. Some people grow up 'touch hungry'—desperate for someone to hold them, to make them feel they exist in their emptiness. On a less extreme level, you may know of folk in your church who would rather not shake hands—they dislike touch, and recoil from physical closeness.

What has all this to do with breastfeeding? When a baby is fed and held and loved constantly by his parents then he will grow up knowing he is valued, confident in himself as a loved, lovable person, able to touch and to be touched, and perhaps later, a daughter becomes a mature mother, to breastfeed her own children with that same devotion. If all babies had this warm, human experience at the breast, how much healthier our children would be, physically, emotionally and spiritually.

When we look at Jesus as a baby and as a mature man, it is not only what we see in him, but what we bring *to* him from our experience that becomes an experience of truth. God's love then 'rings bells' deep within our minds and hearts and we can know with certainty that that love is for us and for our families and friends. A desolate, empty start to life and relationships can so easily result in our believing God is empty and demanding. Total disbelief may be the only defence for our already injured minds. Once we can begin to understand why we cannot see or feel love, then we can turn to God in our disbelief and ask him by his grace to soften our hardness, fill our emptiness, and help us to see the glimmer of hope which heralds a new experience of him. There is no need to ask him to love us—he already does, just as an adoring mother looks upon her baby as she feeds him. God supplies all our needs—physical, emotional and spiritual—as a good mother supplies all her child's needs. It is not too late for us to be as little children, and to rest in his arms, and allow the light of his countenance to shine upon us.

When I was a child I talked like a child,
I thought like a child, I reasoned like a child.
When I became a man,
I put childish ways behind me.

Now we see but a poor reflection;
Then we shall see face to face.

Now I know in part;
Then I shall know fully, even as I am fully known.

And now these three remain:
Faith, hope and love.
But the greatest of these is love.

1 Corinthians 13:11-13
New International Version

Lord Jesus, giver of life and health,
We thank you that our babe
Grows strong, happy and free.
May your continued blessings flow
So that we may radiate your love in
our lives.
Thank you for the privilege and joy
Of caring for and feeding this child.
We pray that as our baby grows
He/she may be filled with
The power of the Holy Spirit.
Father, all things come from you
And of your own do we give you. Amen.

CHAPTER NINE

Evenings of Tearfulness

A family affair
Grandparents
Naïve needs
Postnatal depression
Into thy hands
Prayer

Childbirth may be one of life's happiest and most fulfilling experiences. A young couple may discover new depths of love and tenderness, care and prayer together. As they adore their baby, they may feel a more powerful expression of God and his love for them than ever before. They begin the adventure of bringing their child up in the joyful anticipation of God's continuing care and commitment, and with loving support given by family, friends and church, are able to rededicate their lives and their baby to his greater glory.

Yet 'mornings of joy give for evenings of tearfulness': for some mothers all does not run so smoothly. A mother today may be depicted in advertisements or on television as being a healthy, glowing, fashionable, bright-eyed, loving mother. Surrounded by expensive toys, soft babywear and with her devoted handsome husband beside her, she holds her cherubic baby—plump, pink and perfect. They are all smiling. They seem to be saying to the young mother: 'This is motherhood today, and if you don't live up to this picture, you are failing.' Sometimes it seems as if a young woman is expected to pause briefly from her career, proceed radiantly through her pregnancy, then quickly, quietly and conveniently give birth to a baby who doesn't cry. Then she returns home to look after Baby, husband and house, and within a month or two continues with her career—her figure and emotions all 'back to normal'. The whole event is simply looked upon as a happy hiccup in her life.

A family affair

In many unindustrialized societies pregnancy and birth is a family affair. Pregnancy is interpreted as fertility, and this adds status and meaning to the girl's life. She may be involved with rituals and rites observed by family, friends and villagers to protect her and her unborn baby from harm. She will have been brought up to regard pregnancy and birth as a normal part of family life, and will be familiar with all it involves. She will have grown up with brothers and sisters, old and young, and she will know how to handle her baby after the birth. Her anxieties and fears, hopes and joys, will be shared with and catered for by the community in which she lives. While she is in labour she will be held, supported, massaged and encouraged by other women—her mother, midwife and aunts or sisters. She will be free to move to any position she feels will help her to give birth more quickly and comfortably. As the baby is born she will quite naturally take and hold him. She will be free to explore the little infant with her fingers—touching, soothing, stroking and caressing. The baby will feed whenever he wants, and may fall asleep at the breast. Held close, the baby lives with his mother as one symbiotic unit. Feeding, rocking as mother moves, hearing her heartbeat and her voice, he gradually widens his horizons and explores the home, always able to return to his mother. If mother is not there for any reason, grandparents or aunts will automatically take over the role of mother. The price paid for this natural family birth is the lack of sophisticated technology to help a mother with an obstructed labour, and in some families babies do not survive the birth and there is mourning and grief within the family as they share the sad experience.

In our western 'civilized' society, there has been a real danger that modern technology would not only cause some obstetric problems, but also seriously interfere with the relationship between the mother and her baby. The often male obstetrician has decided for women what they should or should not experience in their labours, and in the name of safety have sometimes robbed the mother and her baby of the enriching experience birth should be. The dangers arose when new methods of controlling labour were used, not only to rightly save the life of some babies and mothers, but were also used on nearly all mothers as a matter of routine 'just in case' there might be a problem. Women had to lie flat on their backs to give birth, it became fashionable to induce most labours and an episiotomy was routine. Babies were whisked away from Mother so they could sleep in the nursery and be 'free from infection'. Breastfeeding was thought to be rather primitive and something 'nice' middle-class ladies didn't do. Bottle feeds with artificial milk were given four-hourly to babies, to teach them a routine and to begin the process of discipline.

Now, at last, and thank God, things are changing, and doctors are beginning to realize how vital it is for a mother to be left to deliver naturally unless of course there is a serious problem. The importance of the emotional wellbeing of the mother, father and baby has also been realized and the father's presence is now welcomed at the birth in most hospitals. Babies are usually left beside Mother in the hospital, if she wishes, and it is now thought better for them to breastfeed, although babies are still being given occasional bottles of dextrose or milk against parents' wishes in some hospitals. Once home, there may be good or poor support from grandparents, and likewise from health visitors. Our society does not often make provision for paid leave from work for the father.

Great strides have been made in recent years, not only in more advanced technology to help in the case of complicated pregnancies and labours, but also in the realization that Mother, Father and Baby often do far better when a natural birth is encouraged. Good bonding of Mother and Baby in the first hours and days is now recognized as being vital for the future health and happiness of the whole family unit. These changes have occurred largely as a result of women speaking up for themselves, fathers quietly insisting on their rights, and great childbirth educators such as Sheila Kitzinger, Michael Odent and Frederick Leboyer, spreading an enlightened message by their research and writings. We have a lot to be thankful for, but still some way to go.

Grandparents

Our present grandparents and great grandparents were brought up not only with the constant threat of war and hardship, but with much that we now recognize as being poor in midwifery, obstetrics and child care. It must be confusing for them now to see pregnancy and birth treated so differently, and some may feel sad or troubled that they were led to believe that bottle feeding, and a four-hourly routine was the only right way to rear an infant.

In some societies, and especially in parts of the East, grandparents are the most experienced and revered people in the family. They will advise mothers and grandchildren and stand in as surrogate mother if need be. Above all, their wisdom is respected. These days in western society grandparents are sometimes thought of as little more than ex-mothers and fathers who have outmoded ideas, and who are a liability when left with the young! Because of the mobility of our society, grandparents may live many miles away, and consequently only visit the nuclear family at times of celebrations or funerals, only to discover a friction with their daughter or son-in-law as conflicting views on handling the baby emerge.

Our grandparents need to understand how the whole concept of birth and child care has changed. They can be immensely supportive and helpful to their daughter after the birth of a grandchild. I believe it is important to wait until invited, and to keep the length of stay flexible, so that a night or a fortnight—whichever is best for the new parents—will be possible without causing tension or embarrassment. A new mother is quite rightly very possessive of her new baby. When grandparents hold her baby, she may worry that he is anxious, or that he might pick up an infection. I feel it is best if grandparents can help with household tasks and shopping, rather than handle the baby too much. Once the new mother is feeling less vulnerable and less anxious, she may be pleased to allow grandparents to take a fuller role.

Above all, grandparents can be a wonderful emotional strength and support. A new mother and father need to be praised and encouraged, and need

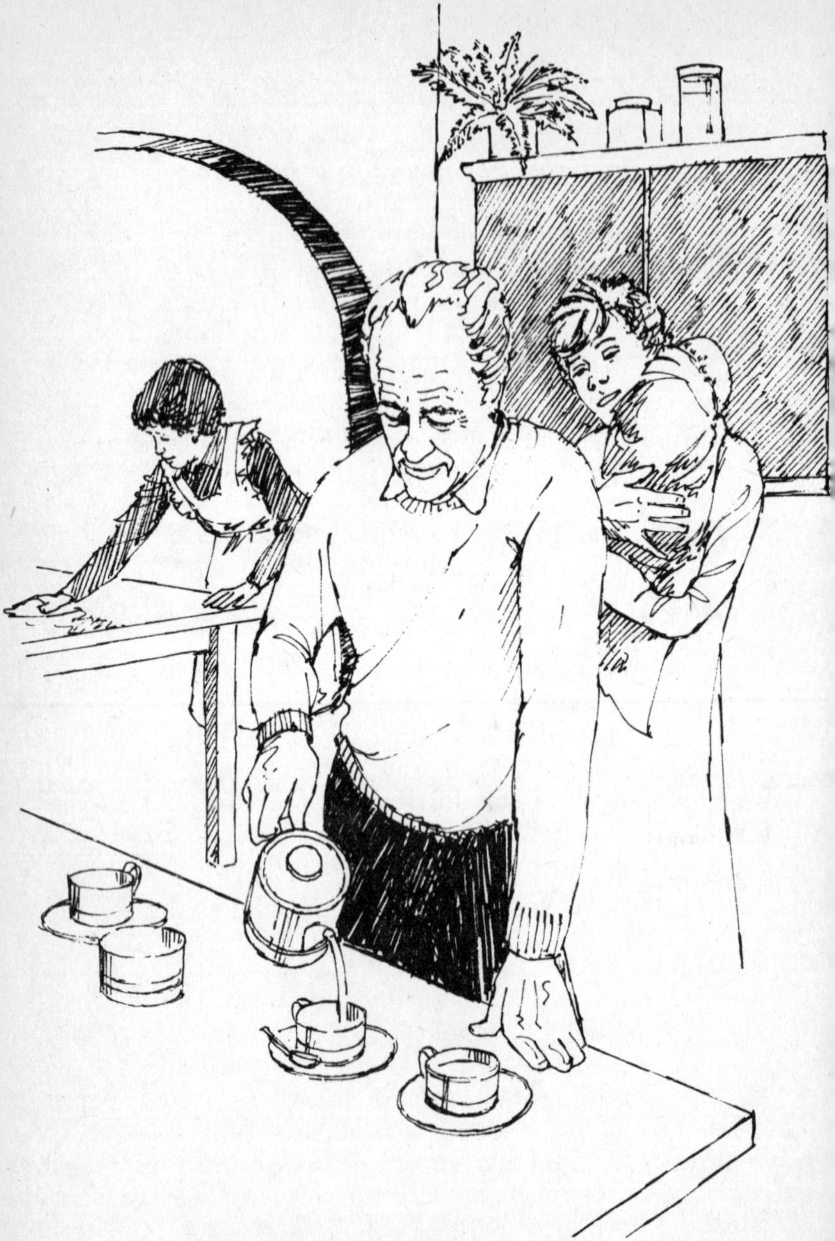

It is best if grandparents can help with household tasks and shopping, rather than handle the baby too much.

to be told they are good parents. They should never have their confidence undermined even in the slightest detail. An arm to give a hug of encouragement, and a shoulder to cry on may be exactly what is needed. A critical eye may destroy confidence and spoil a trusted relationship. 'A kiss for grandma' can be a desperate plea of an empty grandmother needing love for herself, rather than for a toddler. A toddler who is made to feel confident and loved will probably run up to his grandma and give her a kiss anyway! Being a grandparent should not give an automatic passport to babysitting—that is a privilege that needs to be won through love and respect.

Naïve needs

Some of the best tears a couple may shed are the tears of wonder, joy and utter exhaustion which may come immediately after their precious baby is born. The moist flushed skin of your faces may caress the wet wrinkled greasy skin of your baby and your tears mingle with the new sweetness of birth. It is quite usual for Dad to weep with you—such is the overwhelming power of love. Over the coming days you may feel extremely sensitive and open to every emotion; so tired and vulnerable that tears and laughter are never far away. There are many reasons for this, and all are quite natural and understandable. You are very tired. Your body has undergone a sudden rather drastic drop in the level of progesterone (one of the hormones of pregnancy). The impersonal routine of the hospital may upset you. You may feel very nervous about handling your baby, and on top of this you will be coping with lactating breasts and a leaking vagina!

To dismiss tears in these days as being 'just your

hormones' is not only unfair but almost callous. You are likely to feel better once you can be at home with your husband, learning together how to feed, change and hold your baby, free from the potentially critical eyes of professionals! If you are unhappy in hospital, do ask, and get your husband to ask, if you can go home. You need peace and quiet. To feel upset in hospital is hardly conducive to rest. If on the other hand you find your stay in hospital a welcome and happy break from your usual work at home, especially if you have older children, then indulge yourself and make the most of it!

Once you are home, you may both need to adjust to one another as you assume the new roles of Mother and Father. Remember you are both tired, you've both waited through nine months, you've both been busy having the baby, and now you are both disturbed by night feeds and the general upheaval that caring for a new baby entails. You can be of enormous mutual support as you enjoy these special early days. Yet a tiny remark or criticism can seem too harsh—even teasing can be hurtful and what was meant to be a joke can result in tears. Be gentle with one another and you will discover a delightful mutuality in your love and a tenderness which transcends words; it is the Spirit of Christ in your home and in your hearts. Gradually as you feel more rested and more confident, and as the experience of birth fades a little in your minds, you may become stronger, and more able to cope with the everyday ups and downs of life. Your midwife should call each day until the tenth day and hopefully she will reassure you about any anxieties with Baby and check that you are physically returning to normal. If you need any advice concerning breastfeeding, it is best to seek it from one person, rather than a few, as conflicting opinions are so easily given. A local National Childbirth Trust breastfeeding counsellor will be pleased to help at any time, day or night.

Keep talking to one another about your feelings and allow time for each other. It is so easy to get submerged with the nappies or the feeding and suddenly to find you have lost contact with that special naïve part of each other; the part that will need or give a hug, need or give a shoulder to cry on. I like to call it 'naïve need', because it is childlike, simple, and holds no defences against true feelings. It is sometimes easier to get angry, depressed, manic or sexual, rather than to admit it is a naïve need, a child-like holding, love and support that is needed.

Once your husband returns to work, you may become more dependent on friends or neighbours for help and support. Most people will rally round when they know there's a new baby, and soon you will find yourself pushing the baby out in a pram, as proud as punch! If you can mix with other new mums you will be able to share ideas and feelings. The National Childbirth Trust has a postnatal support organization in each area which offers friendship and mutual support over coffee which can make all the difference to you. It is easy to feel lonely with your baby, and when you are physically tired with broken nights and busy days you may become depressed.

Postnatal depression

Postnatal depression is an illness, a pathological state. It affects one mother in every ten—that's a lot of mothers—and those are only the reported cases.

Some mothers start to feel depressed on or around the third day after delivery—this is often called the 'baby blues'—and, as we have already discussed, it is an understandable and natural condition. It only becomes abnormal if it fails to pass, clamping the new mother in a type of miserable depersonalized haze. Occasionally there may be little or no sign of depression until two or three weeks after the delivery, or even two or three months.

If this happens to you, you may feel very unhappy, anxious, tired, and trapped in a feeling of unreality. Baby may seem distant or even remote, and you may be unsure whether you love the baby or not, or feel that you can't express your love. Some mothers feel like a machine that changes nappies, feeds and cleans. Soon you may begin to feel acute guilt that you are not the bright, smiling, confident mother your friends and family expect you to be. Night feeds can be a special agony. Heavy with sleep, you feed the baby who seems to drain you of your very self. You long to sleep and feel acutely lonely. You may cry bitterly and be quite unable to find the 'real you' through this depression.

Husband, family and friends may not realize for some time that you are really depressed. People expect a new mother to be a bit 'emotional' and put it down to their being tired, or to their 'hormones'. Even your health visitor or doctor may make similar comments and pass your complaint of depression over with a quick reassuring phrase. It's not that people don't care, but depression in a new young mother somehow goes against the grain of our expectations. It threatens people and makes them feel anxious and rather inadequate. It is a bit like bereavement.

If you are feeling depressed, do try and talk to your partner about how you feel. Wait and see how you are in a few days, but don't delay too long before going to see your doctor. If he decides to wait and see how you are the following week, do be sure to keep that second appointment, and if you are no better *ask* for treatment.

The causes of your depression may be many. Your mind and body have been through a crisis—especially if you had a difficult, anxious or painful labour—and you may be reacting to the stress as a type of delayed reactive depression. If this is the case, you may be helped by being prescribed an anti-depressant drug. These drugs are not addictive, but one drawback is that it's two to three weeks before any beneficial effect is felt. In the meantime you may experience some side effects such as a dry mouth, fine tremor or lethargy. However, some mothers respond well to anti-depressant therapy and it may be worth persevering. It is safe to breastfeed while taking these drugs, but make sure your doctor knows.

Another reason for postnatal depression is an inadequate amount of the hormone progesterone. During your pregnancy high levels of this hormone build up in your bloodstream, which is one reason why some mothers feel so healthy and happy during those months. With the expulsion of the placenta, that supply of progesterone is suddenly cut off, and it may be many weeks before the body produces the normal non-pregnant amount again. In the meantime, the sudden deprivation of the hormone may cause a severe and solid depression.

Dr Katharina Dalton has done special research into hormones and their effect on puerperal depression. She has treated mothers by giving them intramuscular injections of progesterone (it cannot be taken in tablet form) over several weeks, with some success. General practitioners in several areas are now understanding more about the importance of progesterone, and are successfully treating mothers with postnatal depression. Unfortunately the drug cannot be synthetically produced, so the drug companies are not advertising it. The drug progestogen is synthetic. It is contained in the pill. Progestogen actually lowers the level of progesterone in the blood so any mother taking the pill may have her depression worsened. Dr Katharina Dalton devotes a chapter to the important difference between progesterone and progestogen in her book *The Premenstrual Syndrome and Progesterone Therapy* (Heinemann Medical Books, 1977).

Occasionally a course of psychotherapy may be of value in the treatment of depression, especially if there are personality or marital problems.

Very occasionally (about one in five hundred), a puerperal or postnatal depression left untreated may become a far more serious puerperal psychosis. This is a state of mind in which the mother may have false beliefs about herself or her family. She may hallucinate and be unable to control her mood, which may fluctuate from stuperose depression to mania. This illness requires urgent medical treatment and some good psychiatric hospitals have mother and baby units where mothers suffering from this distressing illness may be nursed back to normality with staff supervising the care of the baby.

In conclusion, it is vital that a new mother is helped with proper medical treatment if she becomes seriously depressed in the weeks or months following the birth. A quick psychological pat on the back is not enough. Alongside medical treatment, she may need a great deal of help with the baby, and will need comfort and support over the coming months until her mood is normal and she can face the world again with a happy confidence.

Into thy hands

It seems that through the ages some degree of suffering is inextricably bound up with childbirth. Pain is expected and catered for, whether it be in primitive or advanced societies. To suffer in childbirth is almost like an initiation into motherhood. Some women who have missed out on pain or extreme pressure, as in the case of a Caesarean section, or with epidural anaesthesia, have felt cheated of an experience they expected to feel. They have almost disbelieved the baby was theirs. One girl who had an incredibly easy, painless delivery kept saying to me that she couldn't believe she had had a baby, couldn't believe the baby was hers. One wonders in these cases what effect this has on the natural bonding of mother and child. Films or novels describing childbirth usually like to dramatize pain, while our Christian heritage depicts a placid Madonna and Child almost without exception! That a mother's travail is quickly forgotten as she sees her child is true, but the fact that she leaks, feels exhausted and may become depressed is somewhat glossed over.

If there is a comical side to the after effects of childbirth, I'm quite sure God is the first to laugh with us! Sometimes to realize this fact is enough to cheer us up and keep us going through each day's mundane chores. You need to ask God to be with you in all you do and say during those sensitive early days and weeks, and remember—there need be no taboo on tenderness. If you suffer from depression, try to find an experience of God in the darkness and chaos. He is there, in your very unbelief he lovingly waits beside you. He will not bludgeon his way into your mind. He will watch and wait alongside you, until one day you see that faint glimmer of hope. You may see it in a flower, in your husband's love and care for you, or in your baby's smile. From the arid desert of despair will well up the tears of feeling, and you can cry again, and curl up in relationship with him. Your husband may be the only one whose love you can feel; even God's love seems to you to have disappeared. But then you meet Christ in his tenderness and concern for you.

None of us wants to suffer pain, despair and a feeling of rejection and loneliness. Jesus knelt in the Garden of Gethsemane and asked that the cup be taken from him. But it was not to be. He knows what it is to suffer, he understands, he's done it all before us and for us. Once you come through your valley of depression, you may discover that you are a deeper, richer person and that you have a more valuable relationship with your husband and with God. God doesn't send you the depression, but he can enable you to make a precious pearl out of your trouble, like an oyster makes a pearl from a grain of sand, and then your crying days will be over.

Dear Father, we bring before you
Our sensitivity and frailty.
The days are tiring, and tears close by.
We need a heavenly hug, Lord,
So that we may be reminded of
Your great compassion and loving
  kindness.
May we let go and let God—
For your eyes look on us with such
Infinite love, understanding and humour.
Teach us to care and not to care,
And teach us to be still.
For in your will is our peace. Amen.

CHAPTER TEN

The Lord Is His Name

The reality of parenthood
Another baby
Love
Prayer

WITH THE BIRTH of your baby, a new family is born: a new mother, new father and new grandparents. It is a time of change and a time of experimentation in your new capacity and social role. Many young mothers today have had very little or no experience of handling, or even being with, a tiny baby. Fathers may have had even less. There is now a very real need to share your uncertainties, anxieties and delights of discovery with each other. The fantasy of parenthood can be shattered as tiredness and tears blend with the wonders and satisfaction of the reality of parenthood. You are not expected to be perfect parents, your baby will only too soon need to come to terms with the imperfections of this world. You and your baby can learn together to accommodate one another's weaknesses. Mistakes, accidents, wrong decisions and indifference are usually fairly frequent occurrences in a busy home with young children, but we are resilient creatures and, bonded together with plenty of laughter, honest tears, and God's all-encompassing love, we get by. Our parenthood and their childhood is good enough—and that is good!

The reality of parenthood

Throughout your pregnancy you may have formed an imaginary picture of your baby. You may have hoped for a certain type of labour and birth. A newly pregnant girl telephoned me this week wanting to come to antenatal classes. She said she wanted a totally drug-free labour, a Leboyer-type delivery and intended to fully breastfeed her baby. I hope she has all she wants, but my job will be to help her understand why she has such high expectations of herself and her baby, and to bring about a more flexible attitude. During labour and birth your hopes and expectations are being continually modified and altered so as to come to terms with the reality of your experience. You may be amazed that your baby is a girl, when you've expected a boy, staggered that she has lots of dark hair, and relieved she hasn't got your husband's nose! You may have to accept that it was a long hard labour—perhaps you needed help with pain or eventually had a Caesarean section. Breastfeeding was more difficult than you imagined and you are only just coping and feeling pretty low. Parenthood is a learning experience, and learning about our limitations and achievements can bring about a greater maturity in ourselves as people. You may be parents now, but you are still husband and wife, lovers and partners who have committed themselves to each other and to God. The reality of your labour, with its excitements and disappointments, now merges into the daily routine of life with your baby. If you expect too much of yourselves or your baby you may become frustrated and despondent. Bringing up a baby often stirs up memories and feelings from our own childhood. A crying baby can disturb a little part of ourselves that perhaps once cried like that, or which still would like to be able to cry like that. As you comfort your child, so also you need to comfort yourselves and one another, as God comforts you. Sometimes your own inner-child can cope no longer, and you may feel a great rush of anger or even rage towards your crying baby. Most mothers, if they are honest, have felt like this at times. You are not wicked or a failure, you are you, you are human. You have needs as well as your baby. Remorse often follows your anger, and you wonder how you could ever have felt so desperate. If you can manage to make yourself a warm drink, curl up for a while, sigh out your tension, relax and feel cherished by your heavenly Father, you will begin to find peace and love again, and will be able to share this even greater love with your baby.

It may be helpful if you can both talk about the way you expect to bring up your child. You may have come from very different backgrounds and have vastly different attitudes to home life, families and schools. How do you intend to control or discipline your child when, at eighteen months, he may surprise you and throw a temper tantrum in the supermarket? How do you feel about children in church? Should children ever see you having a row? Will you have them vaccinated against whooping cough? You can see that ahead of you lies a minefield of important decisions to be made. To know about each other's attitudes and beliefs will help you to show a united and consistent front and help you to feel confident as parents and in your belief in what is right for your child. You are unique, and what Mrs Bloggs does with her children may be quite different from what you intend to do with yours. You may both be right, just different. As your baby develops, you rejoice in his accomplishments at each stage. The first time he rolls

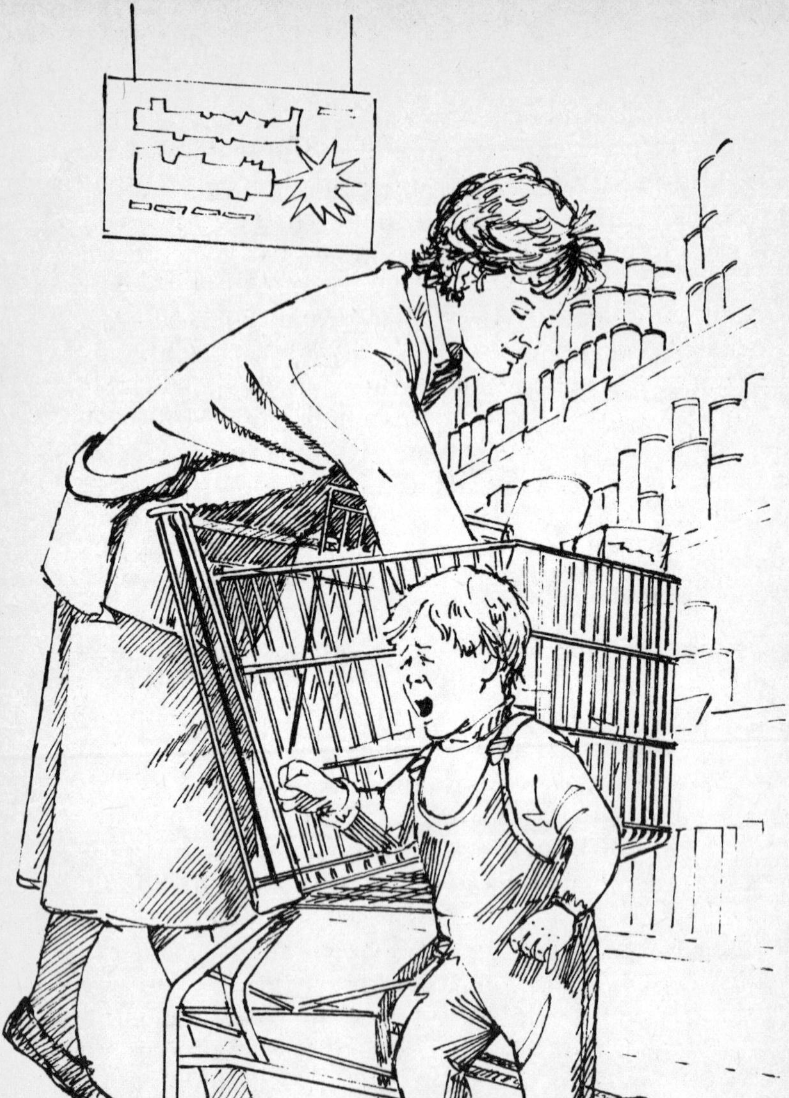

How do you intend to control or discipline your child when at eighteen months he may surprise you and throw a temper tantrum in the supermarket?

over by himself, cuts his first tooth, takes his first step or says those first words are thrilling moments.

New aspects of your personalities will also develop as you comfort your baby after a tumble, get cross with him for being disobedient, smack his hand, or gently encourage him to overcome a fear. There are disappointments too. He may be a baby that cries a lot or sleeps little. He may have eczema or be allergic to cows' milk. He may look like his grandad. He may not speak as soon as others, or may be overactive or rough. Parenthood is a full-time job—physically, emotionally, intellectually and spiritually. One moment your heart aches, then your temper flares or you swell with pride or weep with disappointment. Don't listen to people who say all this will change once you're through the baby stage—my boys are nearly teenagers and life is every bit as full of emotion and hard work! No wonder mothers feel tired at the end of the day and no wonder they can feel immensely fulfilled.

Another baby

You may wonder about another child. The belief that an only child is always overindulged, spoiled and lonely is not borne out by research. Two children are good company for each other; two children may fight. The arguments are endless—so are the possibilities. Having children close together can be a strain on parents, or it may feel good to 'get it all over with' in a short time. A larger gap between children can help each child to feel special for longer, but would prolong the time you are 'tied' to babies. Obviously there is not one answer. It is simply a matter of what suits you, your home, your energy, your career and your finances.

When you give birth to your second or third child you will need to make special arrangements for the other children. They may be excited about the baby, but have no concept of what it means in terms of you being away for a while, breastfeeding, or being tired. A home birth means that the children could even be present at the birth—perhaps this will be accepted in hospitals before long. When your toddler first comes to see you after the birth of another child, I believe that first and foremost your child wants to be reassured that you still love him—the new baby is almost incidental to this. If you can have the new baby in a cot across the room and have your arms free to give toddler a big hug, it may be less threatening to him than if your arms are full with the new baby, or you are feeding him. A secure, loved toddler, confident in his mother's love can then venture out to discover the new baby for himself rather than having a brother or sister thrust at him, then be expected to love them. To a toddler, the addition of a new baby may feel like a loss, and there may be sorrow in the child. He has lost the special relationship the first child enjoys with his parents. He has lost that total devotion, he no longer has toys to himself. He may show his sorrow by trying out ways of regaining that unique relationship—so demanding extra time and attention from Mother, or smacking the new baby. These need to be controlled, but all seem quite sensible really when you understand what toddler is trying to say. He will learn to enjoy baby and share his home once he is absolutely sure the new baby isn't going to lessen his parents' love for him. He will need to learn to share and this can be painful, but he can also discover the delight of being big brother and of helping mother, and having a playmate with whom to enjoy life.

If you do intend to have another baby, you may need to realize that each pregnancy, labour and birth are unique. Whatever you experienced the first time may or may not occur again, whether good or bad. Your body needs to be fully recovered from the first birth. You may find labour is quicker the second time, especially the second stage, as your pelvis will have widened a little after the first delivery, so it may be easier for the next baby to be born. It is wise to go to antenatal classes again at your local hospital as it is surprising how much you may have forgotten about pregnancy and birth, and all the time hospital procedures, attitudes and staff are changing. It is well to be up to date and knowledgeable about the latest possibilities in childbirth. The National Childbirth Trust run shortened refresher courses in some areas, but the full course may be most beneficial.

If for any reason you need to be away from your first child for any length of time, it is vital that he has someone, perhaps his father, grandmother, aunt or neighbour, who is able to give the same consistent love and care he has been used to. Perhaps a problem in your pregnancy might necessitate a lengthy stay in hospital, or some problem with the health of the new baby might mean you need to be away from home. This is very stressful for all of you, but most of all for a toddler who cannot understand the situation. Children may feel they have done something wrong for Mother to leave them or that they are bad. At first, without a good substitute mother, there is protest that you have gone, accompanied by tears and temper. Gradually protest turns into despair—there seems to be no point in creating a fuss. Thirdly, if the separation is protracted, there comes detachment, a state of unrelatedness to anyone and a dislocation from their own emotions. This could lead to life-long pain at the separation with possible neurotic or even psychotic behaviour. Thankfully it is usually the case that someone 'good enough' cares for the child and some form of protest is the worst that ever happens. If you do have to leave your toddler, even for a short time, try to understand that if the child is angry when you return, or even rejects you he may be expressing his sense of anger at being left. He may need time to realize you really are back and that he need protest or despair no more. If you rush to hold and hug him it may frighten him. He needs to rediscover your love for him gently and gradually, and rebuild his trust in you.

Love

This book has been about pregnancy and childbirth, but it has also been about love. You have been on a kind of love journey. It began with learning to love yourselves, to prepare yourselves lovingly during pregnancy, to love each other through the birth experience. You have looked at the possibility of losing love and of discovering a greater love in depths of darkness. You have seen the love of God shining in and on your baby's face, bringing you comfort if depressed.

But what exactly is love? We use the word 'love' each day in some context. 'I'd love to go for a walk'; 'I love you'; 'You are a love'; 'It's a lovely day.' We are familiar with the word from our earliest days. Yet love is an experience, not a part of speech. It holds for us deep meaning, and for each of us the significance and experience of the word will be different.

Sometimes you may need love, sometimes you may give love. Love has a powerful physical effect on us. As babies, a loving hold, eyes and smile all tell us that we mean something good. We are valued and cherished. Physically it gives us a feeling of wellbeing. Loved babies thrive. Their eyes shine, they respond delightfully to loving people, and soon learn to copy them. They put on weight, stay healthy and grow. A baby totally unloved and unstimulated will withdraw into himself, will not develop, will cease to feed, will fail to thrive and will die. Love has a drawing-together quality. People want to be with the one they love and dislike separation. Love seeks out closeness and encourages commitment to one another. Being together in marriage brings the ultimate union of sexual intercourse, of making love and all that this expresses. When we are in love, our hearts ache with love. A mother will know physically that her baby needs her, and a breastfeeding mother will leak milk at the thought of her baby's needs. Love seems to be a mixture of pleasure and pain, as though we need the one to balance the other. Watching a child take a new step further in life brings the pleasure of success and the pain of loss. Watch how you feel as your toddler goes to playschool for the first time. Letting love go is painful, but brings its rewards.

Throughout the ages, writers, poets and musicians have tried to express a language of love. Yet there are no words adequate, for love is the experience of wonder, of mystery. Love is incomprehensible to us, too great a mystery. Too good to be true. I believe that love is from God, for God is love. Only perfect love in God can show us the 'how much moreness' of love. We can find God's love in our love for our children, our partners, in all the joys of our relationships. We can find God's love in the beauty and sensuous delight of his creation and in the power and force of nature. We discover that even in the darkness of despair, loss, grief and pain, there is God. Yet God is not 'just out there'. He is to be found deep in our minds and souls. He comes up from the depths and enables us to love himself, others and ourselves.

Why I am so concerned about love is that I believe babies first see love, learn about and experience love, and God, primarily through their mothers and fathers. This good, positive affirmation of the self goes with them throughout their lives, growing and maturing through relationships, physically, emotionally and spiritually, enabling them to discover a richness and a peace in this world and a certain experience of the love of God in their lives. Loving incorporation into a human family is a necessary meaningful prelude to the loving incorporation into the family of Christ. When they later meet with God in Christ they have an experience with which to compare and contrast his love that passes understanding.

He is the Lord, and his name is Love.

For the gift of this child
We praise you, heavenly Father.
Prepare us for the task that lies ahead,
In our weariness, help us to rest,
In our decisions, stay close by.
When tears fall, or tempers flare,
Show us the funny side of things.
Cherish and guide our new family, Lord,
So that we may know you more clearly,
Love you more dearly,
And follow you more nearly,
Our merciful Redeemer.
Amen.

Some Further Reading

G. Lux Flanagan, *The First Nine Months of Life* (Heinemann Medical, 1963).

Pregnancy and Parenthood (National Childbirth Trust, OUP).

Sheila Kitzinger, *Pregnancy and Birth* (Michael Joseph, 1980).

Sheila Kitzinger *The Experience of Childbirth* (Gollancz, 1972).

Sheila Kitzinger, *Women as Mothers* (Fontana).

Susan Borg & Judith Lasker, *When Pregnancy Fails* (RKP).

Máire Messinger, *The Breastfeeding Book* (Century).

Sheila Kitzinger, *The Experience of Breastfeeding* (Penguin, 1979).

Frederick Leboyer, *Birth Without Violence* (Fontana, 1977).

Janet & Arthur Balaskras, *New Life—The Exercise Book for Childbirth* (Sidgwick & Jackson, 1984).

Harry Williams, *True to Experience* (Mitchell Beasley, 1984).

Useful Addresses

The National Childbirth Trust
9 Queensborough Terrace
London
W2 3TB
01 223 3833

The Compassionate Friends
25 Kingsdown Parade
Bristol
0272 47316

Parents Anonymous
9 Manor Gardens
Islington
London
N7
01 263 8918

Society to Support Home Confinements
c/o Margaret Whyte
17 Laburnum Avenue
Durham City
0385 61325

The Stillbirth Association
15a Christchurch Hill
London
NW3 1JY
01 794 4601

Dr Dobson Answers Your Questions about Raising Children

by James Dobson

Dr James Dobson is highly respected as a leading expert on human psychology and Christian family life. Over the years he has been asked hundreds of questions, and this book sets out the answers he has given on a wide range of issues that affect the growth of the individual and the value of family life.

In *Raising Children* Dr Dobson gives practical insights on—

- quality family time
- spiritual training
- the learning process
- sex education
- discipline
- sibling rivalry
- hyperactivity
- adolescence

James Dobson is President of Focus on the Family, a charitable body dedicated to the preservation of the home. For fourteen years he was Associate Clinical Professor of Pediatrics at the University of California School of Medicine, and was appointed by Presidents Jimmy Carter and Ronald Reagan to advise on family and juvenile matters. He is married with two children.

The contents of this book previously appeared in *Dr Dobson Answers Your Questions*.

k Kingsway Publications

Dare to Discipline

by James Dobson

The chaos which reigns in many schools, and even homes, today shows only too clearly the need for practical guidance in disciplining children and young people.

Dr Dobson, a Christian psychologist, spells out the dangers of adopting unworkable permissive theories, recently popular but resulting in increasing disenchantment, and explains the biblical principles for creating respect and responsibility in young people: a balanced approach to discipline, far from inhibiting a child's growth, provides the secure framework within which these qualities can develop.

Over 2,260,000 copies sold.

Discipline while you can

by James Dobson

To those who have never experienced parenthood the job may appear simple, but those of us who are involved know that it is more difficult than it looks.

Children are costly in time and effort, as well as financially—but they are certainly worth the price. This book shows us how to cope with the difficulties and how to train the child who is strong-willed and assertive.

Dr James Dobson, author of the best-seller *Dare to Discipline*, writes with warmth and humour about the problems of infancy, childhood and adolescence, about childhood rivalry and hyperactivity—and deals, too, with the most common errors made by frustrated parents.

Kingsway Publications